Praise for

The Herb Lover's Spa Book

"Here is your formula for relaxation. From sanctuary spaces to growing a garden of fragrant herbs, expert herbalist Sue Goetz inspires you to pamper yourself with gifts from the garden. Sue shares a bounty of recipes that use common herbs and everyday ingredients to create fragrant, luxurious spa treatments. You may never have to pay for spa services again!"

~ Debra Prinzing, author of *Slow Flowers*

"In a fast paced, work-driven life, relaxation is a luxury, an indulgence that seems almost sinful to admit. *The Herb Lover's Spa Book* gives us permission to enjoy a little pampering. By revealing many unique ways to incorporate a sense of spa into our home and garden, Sue Goetz encourages us to find a health-promoting, nurturing balance in our lives once again."

~ Karen Chapman, Le Jardinet garden design, co-author of *Fine Foliage*

"The garden as spa? Who knew? Sue's written a fantastic book featuring her favorite herbs and recipes for using them to create heavenly soaks, teas, elixirs, rubs and more. The recipes are my favorite part of the book, and new "go-to" spa experience. Make plenty of these deliciously fragrant treats for yourself – or for gifts."

~ Mary Ann Newcomer, The Dirt Diva, author and radio host

"Sue will take you away into a world of soothing herbal renewal. From flavorful herbal teas to refreshing facials, learn how your garden holds the secrets of the spa experience. You don't need to be a gardener to appreciate the wisdom of adding herbs to your life."

~ Marianne Binetti, writer, speaker, TV host and author of 10 gardening books, including *Herb Gardening for Washington and Oregon*

"Gardeners know gardening is good for the mind, body and spirit. Sue helps us take it one step further with her new book: putting those plants we love to grow to work, helping us relax and luxuriate. She includes recipes for creating your own spa treatments and inspiration to create your own home spa. And best of all, her approach makes it easy for all to achieve."

~ Melinda Myers, author, TV and radio host, horticulturist and gardening expert

"In *The Herb Lover's Spa Book*, Sue Goetz shares how to slow down and harness the healing powers of the garden to pamper ourselves – something incredibly valuable and often overlooked. Through her clear tutorials and step-by-step recipes, she shares the value in these amazing little plants and how we can use them to rejuvenate ourselves every day."

~ Theresa Loe, Co-executive TV Producer & Canning/Homesteading expert on PBS's "Growing a Greener World"

"Take a deeeeeep breath…now relax. How many times have you gone to get a massage, facial or even a hair treatment and as you are getting that fabulous pampering, you wonder why you don't do this every week? Well, now YOU will have the inside secrets for not only creating a landscape where you can grow the beautiful and useful plants that go into those treatments, but you can learn the magical salon tips for making your own luxurious products. Sue Goetz is a wonderful guide."

~Christina Salwitz, The Personal Garden Coach and co-author of *Fine Foliage*

"As a fellow herb lover, I'm inspired to learn more ways to use a variety of herbs, especially to create my own heavenly herbal spa. Sue's strong gardening background, along with her down-to-earth approach, has created a bounty of herbal spa possibilities – all from easy-to-grow plants with straight-forward directions. *The Herb Lover's Spa Book* is brimming with enticing, luscious and restorative herbal treatments."

~ Beth Evans-Ramos, blogger, "Mama Knows Her Cocktails"

The Herb Lover's Spa Book

The Herb Lover's Spa Book

Create a Luxury Spa Experience at Home
with Fragrant Herbs from Your Garden

Sue Goetz

st. lynn's
press

PITTSBURGH

The Herb Lover's Spa Book
Create a Luxury Spa Experience at Home with Fragrant Herbs from Your Garden

ISBN-13: 978-0-9892688-6-8

Library of Congress Control Number: 2014944844 . CIP information available upon request

First Edition, 2015

St. Lynn's Press . POB 18680 . Pittsburgh, PA 15236 . 412.466.0790 . www.stlynnspress.com

Book design – Holly Rosborough • Editor – Catherine Dees

PHOTO CREDITS:
Photo on p. 170 courtesy of Hayley Goetz. All other photos courtesy of the author and Courtney Goetz.

LINE ART:
p. xx: 1,001 Floral Motifs and Ornamentals for Artists and Craftspeople, Dover Publications, Inc., 2013;
pps. 32 and 56: 200 Illustrations from Gerard's Herbal, Dover Publications, Inc., 2005; p. 36: Karen Watson,
www.thegraphicsfairy.com, re: 1890's Pharmacy catalog; p. 78: public domain, source unknown.

DISCLAIMER:
This book is intended for personal use and not to diagnose a medical condition. All recipes and information are researched for their safe ingredients and are used for topical preparation only, unless specifically noted as a beverage All of the herbal information is sourced from reputable research and author's personal experience and regarded as safe. Not all claims are approved or advised for use by the FDA.

The healing qualities and recipes in this book are not for internal consumption unless specifically noted. Always use any ingredient, even in its raw, natural state with caution on sensitive and allergy-prone individuals, babies and persons with medical conditions. The recommendations for spa treatments are not intended for use by pregnant or nursing women.

The recipes and mix of ingredients presented in this book are researched and tried and created for personal use. They were developed through the author's experiences, practice and knowledge base. Any similarities of recipes or outcome with other works printed or otherwise are purely coincidental.

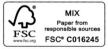

Printed in Canada on certified FSC recycled paper
using soy-based inks

MIX
Paper from
responsible sources
FSC® C016245
www.fsc.org

This title and all of St. Lynn's Press books may be purchased for educational,
business, or sales promotional use. For information please write:
Special Markets Department . St. Lynn's Press . POB 18680 . Pittsburgh, PA 15236

10 9 8 7 6 5 4 3 2 1

To my girls:

Alyssa, Hayley and Courtney

Growing up, you came through the door after school to smell…
not the baking of cookies or other edible confections,
but a new herbal concoction of some kind. Thank you for
being willing testers of my recipes – accepting them
with all the pungent failures and fragrant successes.

I am grateful for all the years you let me chase
this gardening passion. I am truly blessed.

♥

Dear Reader~

I write this because I love a garden that gives back. Flowers, fragrance, flavor...all of it. A true giving garden is filled with herbs. Discover them. Grab a leaf, rub it, hold it to your nose and breathe in. Voila! That plain, leafy plant becomes so much more when you learn ways to use it. That is what I share with you.

Grow herbs, find sanctuary spaces in your garden and home. Whip up some indulgent recipes and treat yourself to the herbal spa experience. Then it's your turn. Share your home spa experiences, recipes and garden with me. I'd love to hear from you!

Merci, Sue

herbloversspa.com
facebook.com/herbloversspa

▪ TABLE OF CONTENTS ▪

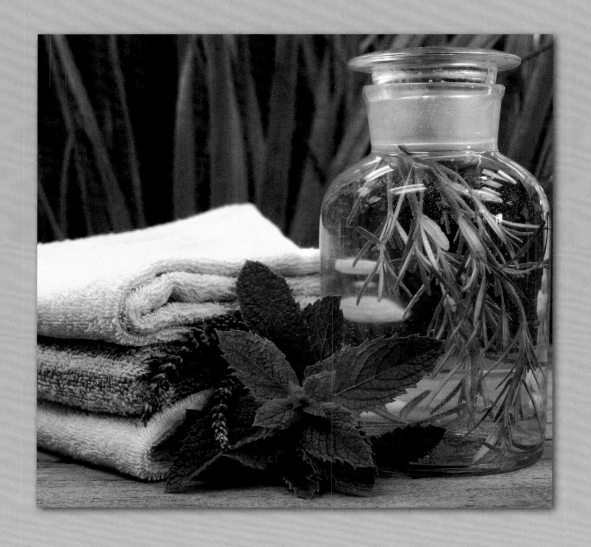

■ INTRODUCTION ■

I am an herb lover, but I am also a spa lover.

When you put the two together, you have the start of

a journey of delight.

"SPA" CONJURES UP SPECIFIC IMAGES FOR ME. A destination resort with fluffy white towels, relaxing massage, luxurious skin treatments and maybe even a fun drink with an umbrella in it. Search online for the word spa and you'll likely find an alluring image of a well-stacked pile of polished black stones next to a candle and a woman with an exotic flower in her hair. Pretty much as expected. But, as I got deeper into writing this book, I become highly aware (with maybe too much sensitivity) of how the word spa is being used for a variety of other commercial purposes – a hot tub company, a pedicure salon, and much more. Recently, I was at a hotel and on the bathroom counter was a row of tiny bottles, each one labeled as a "spa" shampoo, soap, conditioner, bath gel – each one containing a white, silky liquid with no color, no texture. I wondered if it

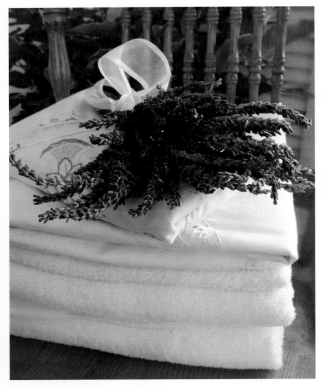

actually use the picture because I have no wish to defame the company that packaged them as "spa" products. But it served as a reminder to me of how generic the word has become.

What is your image of a spa? In the sense of this book, I would like you to visualize the word as a way to nurture and heal. Think of it as a mindset of wellness.

It is all about relaxation in your own surroundings and using herbs from your garden to create a pleasurable, deeply beneficial experience. (Note to those of us who have been treated to a day spa: Creating the spa experience in your own home brings a special degree of relaxation because you don't have to get in the car after your spa day and then drive home afterward. You simply relax, go to bed, meditate or spend moments with renewed energy in your own space. What could be better than that?)

was all the same stuff. I took a picture of the items in the dish and started writing a paragraph in my head with the notion that I needed to debunk this idea of a spa. How dare they? I thought, climbing on my high horse. Of course, I didn't

LESSONS FROM MY GARDEN

My herbal journey began many years ago,

not as a book, but as

lessons from the garden.

Much of my garden learning was in a high mountain desert garden in Idaho. It was in zone 4, and I couldn't grow every herb I wanted to; but oh how I tried! In between killing frosts (usually June and early September) I would grow, gather and preserve as much as possible. In that challenging gardening climate, I used to say if I couldn't make something from the plants, I wouldn't spend my time planting it! I experimented and made many things from the garden; it wasn't always about food, it was also about fragrance and healing.

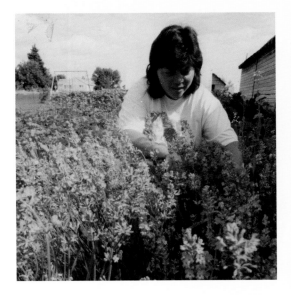

As a garden designer, knowing plants and gardening is what drives my work. I do know that not every plant can be harvested to make something; when I first moved to Washington State, I used to joke about what the heck I can do with a Rhododendron. My work is creating beauty with ornamental plants, but my personal garden passion is all about what the garden gives back.

As a garden speaker, many of my talks are about encouraging people to make discoveries in their own gardens. In recent years, my most requested lectures are about herbs. People are captivated by their fragrance and flavor and all the ways to use them. In 1997, I taught a popular class at the local community college called "Herbal Lotions and Potions." The topic has evolved over time, in both seminar form and as a hands-on workshop – all about growing herbs and using them for skin care.

Then came a discussion with Paul Kelly of St. Lynn's Press and all those lessons, workshops and herbal experiments became the findings for a spa book for herb lovers. During the creation of the book there was an oversized piece of paper posted on the wall of my workspace. In big, black marker I had written the words that I wanted to keep in my thoughts every day:

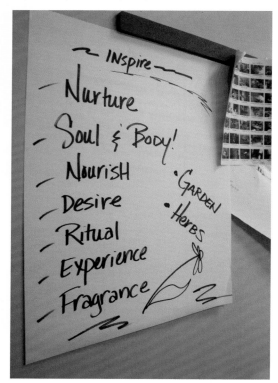

I knew the herbs and recipes by heart, but I wanted to express more, beyond simply making sure you have all the information needed – from the measurement of ingredients to the basics of mixing and blending. I wanted to always find descriptive ways to invite your senses into this herbal journey so you could feel the words, smell the aromas of fresh cut herbs, and anticipate having the comfort of warm healing water touching your skin. I wanted to celebrate the silky

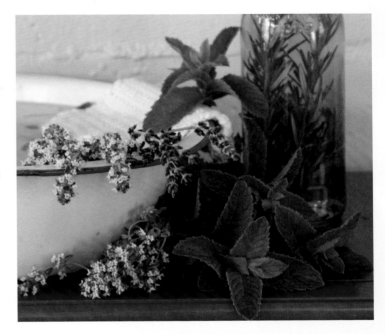

feel of herb-infused grapeseed oil on your hands, and the aroma of just-harvested lemon verbena that elevates your mood just by its fresh fragrance. Do words exist that truly describe the way mint tingles? My answer to myself was: Try as I might to tease and entice, there are just no words that can do full justice to the herbal spa experience itself.

And so I give you my heartfelt invitation to discover for yourself the beyond-words gifts from the herbal garden – your garden – to immerse yourself in the healing qualities of herbs, to care for your body and engage your senses.

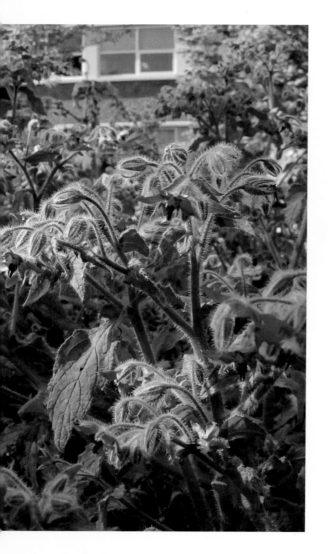

What's Inside

The book is presented in three parts: Surround, Grow and Create.

- **Surround** helps you envision a setting that says ahhh to your soul, much the way a great destination spa can do. This is not about replacing that luxurious experience, it is about capturing it. The destination spa for most of us is a quiet moment in the bathtub. Now go beyond that. Let this part of the book inspire you to create your own personal spa environment – its design, colors and textures – whether it's a private corner of your garden or a place of retreat inside your home, or all of the above.

- **Grow** is about the plants. There are hundreds of plants that are classified as healing herbs, many with excellent qualities to use in spa treatments. For this book, my objective was to keep everything accessible. The list of herbs is small (19), rather than comprehensive. They are common and well known, and they will thrive in a diversity of climates. I want them to be easy for you to grow and use. The recipes in the book use only the 19 herbs I've profiled. (The same goes for other ingredients you'll use in your spa concoctions: recipes using exotic and/or hard to find things were not included. I also stayed away from things that might be risky or have high sensitivity in their interaction with skin and body care.)

Once you have your spa surroundings and your fragrant herbs, it's time to bring it all together.

■ **Create** is about the recipes – lots and lots of them, along with some fun DIY projects. I've put information about ingredients, kitchen tools and preparation right up-front, so you don't have to keep turning to the back of the book to check on something. The recipes are grouped around 11 themes, with names like "Get Steamy" and "The Top-To-Bottom Scrub Experience." The themes are yours to explore and be inspired to experiment with. Plan a romantic evening and use the vanilla infused oil (the Après-Scrub Skin Oil) recipe as a massage oil. Gift friends with homemade scrubs (try Lavender Spa Salt Glow) labeled with a personalized note of encouragement to pamper themselves. Throw a bridal shower and make it a foot spa party (double the recipe for Peppermint Foot Soak) to treat your guests.

■ ■ ■

Please stay in touch about your home spa adventures. Let me know what worked, what didn't, and what you adapted or invented that you'd like to share with others. I hope you enjoy this book!

Warm wishes,

Sue

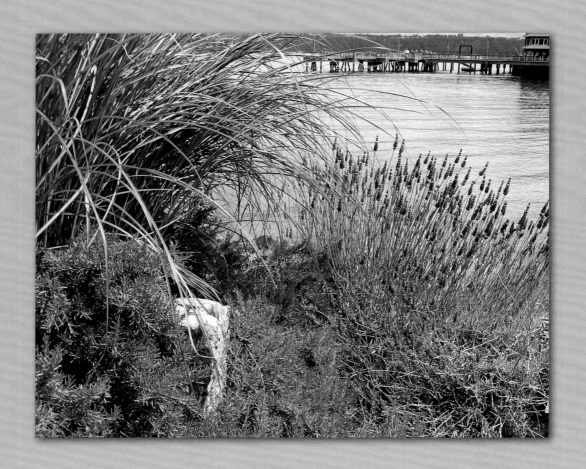

▪ SPA: A LITTLE HISTORY AND LORE ▪

The origin of the word spa is a bit ambiguous. It may have come from the word *espa*, which translates as fountain in the French-Belgian Walloon dialect. Then there is the reputation of the Belgian town of Spa, which is noted as far back as the 1500s, when Henry VIII came there for its healing pools of therapeutic waters… and even before that, when its waters were written about by the 1st century naturalist Pliny the Elder. One way or the other, the word has come down to us as a source of health and pleasure.

"Taking the waters"

All through history, people have been "taking the waters" in places like Spa and around the world – whether it be lounging along the edges of natural earthen pools or enjoying the amenities of elaborate public bathhouses. If you look at the evolution of bathing you will find that cultures everywhere have their own rituals of soaking in water. In the Western world, physicians have long prescribed bathing in waters full of minerals, herbs and other naturally occurring chemicals, to heal whatever one's ailment was. In ancient Greece, bathing was beginning to move from simple hygiene to a communal experience, with bathhouses created for the purpose. Sparta had even developed a kind of steam bath. But it was the Romans who raised the simple ritual of bathing to high art. Roman "thermae" were free public bathhouses used for physical fitness, social interaction and entertainment. They featured heated pools, massage, serene gardens – even libraries. I suspect those waters were awesome therapy, too, for great thinkers to debate global domination while immersed in the steaming water.

In cultures everywhere, we see the many facets of water treatment – from the simplicity of taking a bath in mineral water to full-cleansing, herb-laden therapeutic rituals in beautiful surroundings.

Fragrant herbs and essences

I was interested to discover that those Roman thermae often had perfume shops attached to them. Unlike the modern methods of perfume making (which are usually alcohol-based, with synthetic fragrance added) the ancient foundation of perfumery was based on immersing oneself in natural, aromatic herbs. The use of plants for fragrance dates back to the beginning of historical records, which describe methods of boiling, crushing, pressing and powdering. Plant extracts were used in bathing and for scenting and cleansing linens and clothes, the floors of the home, tiles, tents, horses, and even the sails of ships (more on that in a moment). In Elizabethan times, aromatic herb waters and cut stems of plants were sprinkled on floors to mask unpleasant odors.

As an example of the power of natural scents, consider how Cleopatra chose to use them. We know that she employed wit and charms to get her way in a dangerous world, including the use of precious plant oils. In an attempt to expand her political influence, she seduced Mark Antony by her lavish use of aromatics. Shakespeare, in *Antony and Cleopatra*, described the time when Antony first fell under her spell. There they were, on her magnificent gilded barge: *"Purple the sails, and so perfumed, that the winds were love-sick with them…"*

Value and demand made fragrant plants a commodity on a par with gold and silver. But beyond the fragrance were their treasured healing and nurturing qualities. And so, the ancient power of fragrance and the ritual of healing waters brings us full circle to what we think of as the spa experience: a way to care for the body and soul.

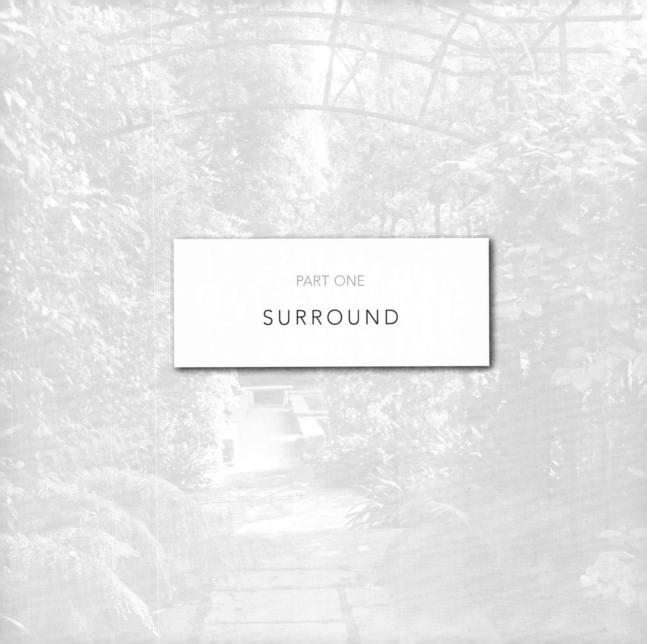

PART ONE

SURROUND

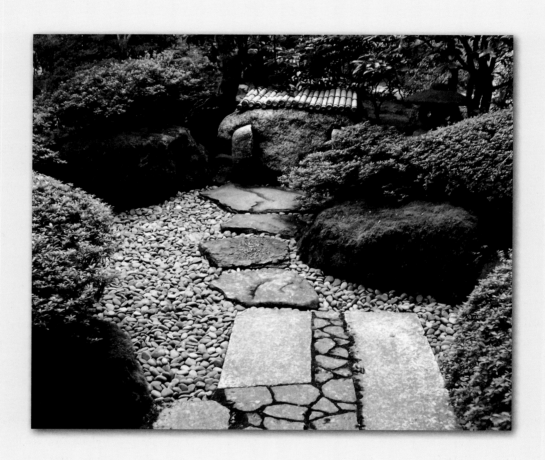

Every person has their "thing"
that helps them relax,

feel cared for and nurtured.

Ask five people what calms them and you will get five different answers. Our complex brain and sensory functions receive outside influence differently. For example, some of us like to have our feet rubbed, while others find it uncomfortable. The same can be said for types of body massage. And when it comes to the power of fragrance, a sense of smell can be so strong that it brings on a headache; yet others of us can hardly recognize the odor of a rose right under our nose. Describe what basil smells like – is it clove-like and warming or reminiscent of tomato sauce poured over pasta? It is all stored in our memory by way of individual experiences. Within those experiences we can also outline what it takes to bring personal relaxation. The creation of your spa experience – the actual space, the sensory stimuli, the mood makers – starts when you truly consider and define what is indulgent and comforting for you.

You might think that the obvious and only place for your personal home spa is the bathroom or hot tub. But, let's expand your idea of a spa and find other spaces that nurture, too – beyond the thought of a bathtub or sink. The relaxing atmosphere can be many places once you have fashioned the surroundings to match your need for refuge and indulgence. It can be indoors, outdoors, or both. Think what it is that relaxes you and discover where that could be. In the pages that follow, we'll look at ways you can create a place that invites you to return again and again.

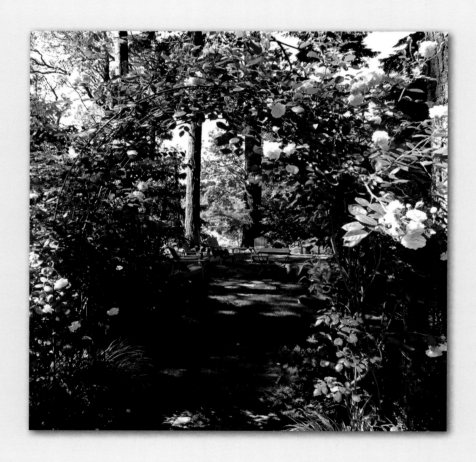

THE GARDEN AS SANCTUARY

As a garden designer, I often hear people say their garden is their therapy. They will work outside in the dark with a flashlight after a long day at work, just to have precious moments to dig in the dirt. It is amazing how a few hours of tending the garden will melt away a whole day of stress. The influence of a garden is written in history and long studied, whether you go back to Eden with Adam and Eve or study the history of medicine derived from plants.

There is much that can be said about how a garden affects us. It all but forces us into a patient tempo and away from the instant gratification that drives so many aspects of modern life. When we're in the garden, there is no device that dings in our

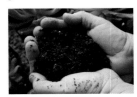

brain when time is up or a computerized sound to remind us to go somewhere. We plant bulbs in dark, damp soil, knowing the fulfillment will be months away. We push tiny seeds into the ground with a memory of the taste of fresh tomatoes off the vine. In the fast-paced life of today, we need to find sanctuary and healing therapy. What is at the top of the list? Planting, nurturing and

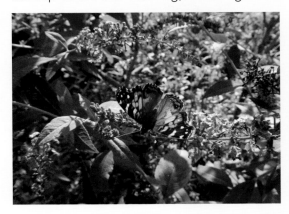

being in the garden. We can toss aside the statistics about the popularity of gardening, and say that it is long-revered as a place to go when one wants to slow down and linger. There is simply something about nature that forces us to not be in a hurry. She is also a powerful seductress that keeps us always longing to smell flowers and gather herbs for tea, and crave the first fresh-picked raspberry.

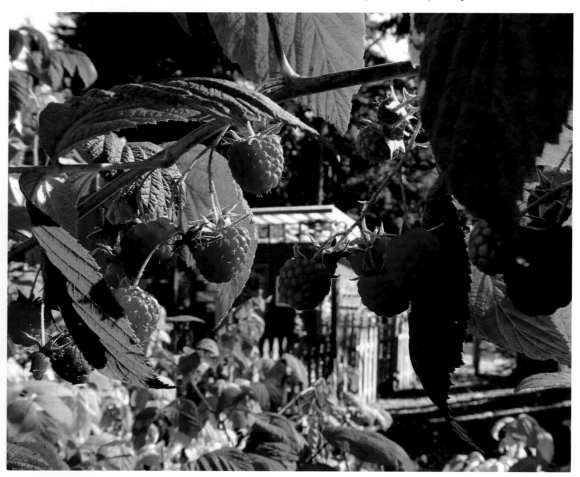

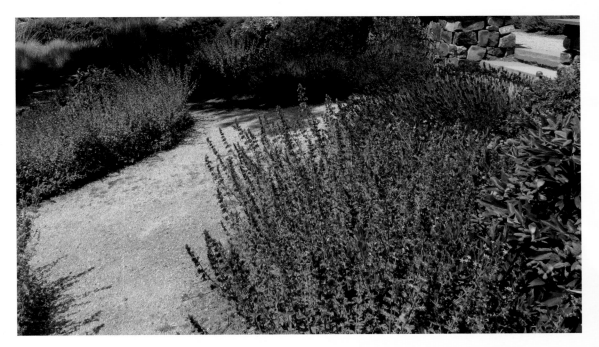

Creating retreat in the garden

Now let's take a walk in a garden that has been planted with herbs and other sensory delights. Slow down and inhale deeply until you feel as if your lungs are filled to capacity, then slowly release your breath. The fresh dose of oxygen runs through you as the earthy fragrances of herbs and flowers weave their way into your mind. Nature's aromatic therapy sends messages to the brain and readies the body for relaxation. The essential oil of some herbs can trigger responses that release calming hormones and slow the rush of adrenaline. (In research studies, lavender essence actually forces a physical response that lowers blood pressure, heart rate and skin temperature.)

Every time we bring ourselves to a place of relaxation the memory preserves it.

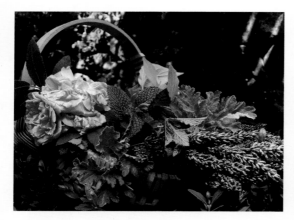

Creating a special space in your garden as a haven will encourage a habit to go there and relax…to jog that relaxation memory all over again. When you go to the next level of making your own spa treatments with fragrant herbs from the garden, your experience will be all the more memorable.

Elements of design

Making a sanctuary space is a very personal project. What says "sanctuary" to you? In a garden it can be the sound of water, a private building for retreat, a rustic pergola, or a collection of favorite plants to sit in the midst of after a busy day. There are no set rules on the actual measurement of space. Large or small in size, it is more about the importance of making it work for you.

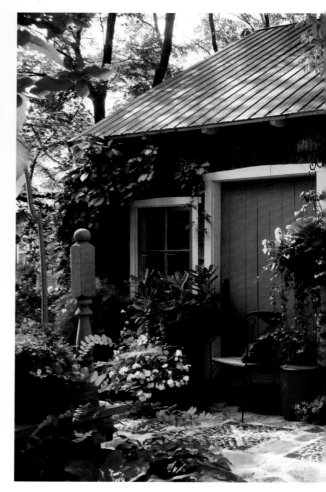

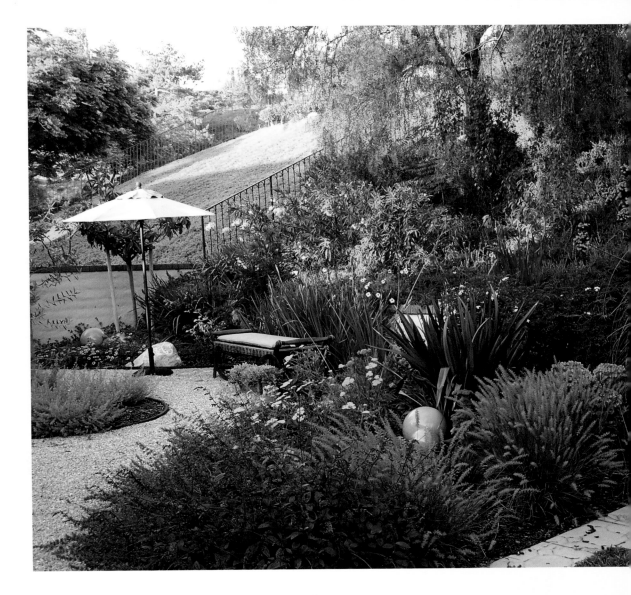

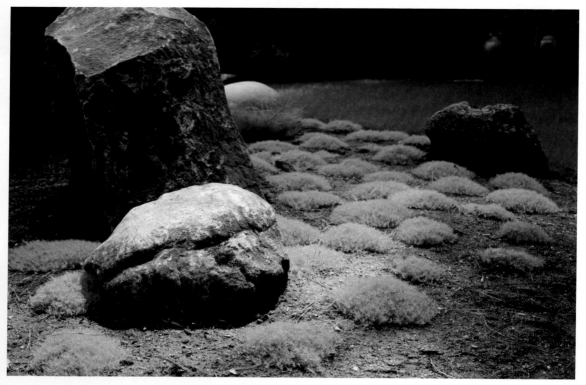

Take a moment to reflect on these words:

TRANQUILITY

Healing

Serenity

Peaceful

Meditation

Calming

ESCAPE

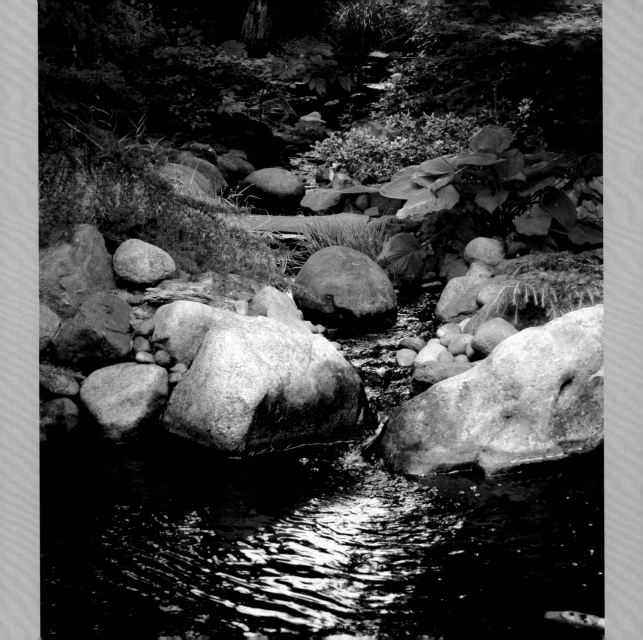

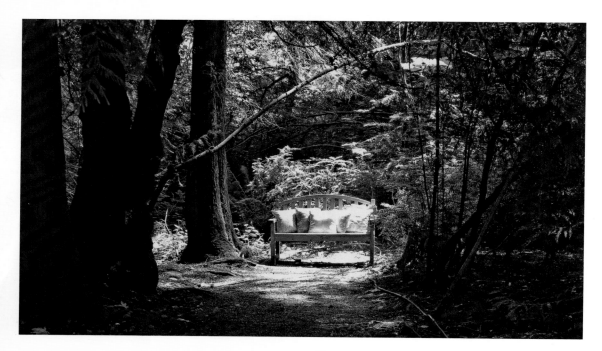

Sanctuary, on an expressive level, is all of these things. The addition of practical pieces of a design will create the privacy, security and comfort you are seeking.

To clarify your planning, start with some questions. The answers will guide you to discover ways of creating a garden sanctuary.

What will I do in the space?

■ *Sleep…eat…read…soak.*

When do I plan on using it most?

■ *In the morning drinking a cup of tea…or evening relaxation after dinner.*

What additions are needed to meet my needs?

- *Reading needs a quiet space with only the gentle, natural sounds of bees humming, splashing water and birds as the backdrop noise.*
- *Sleeping spaces need protection from weather.*
- *For outdoor bathing or showering, privacy is required.*

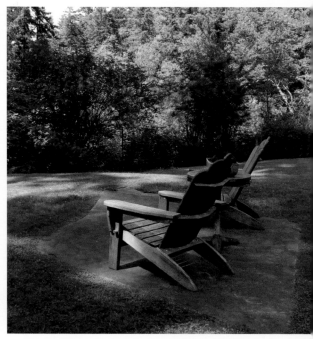

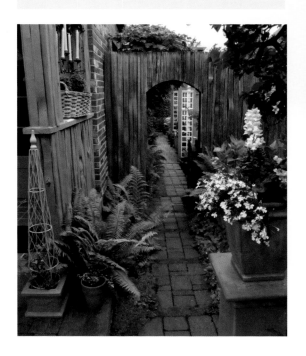

What precludes your enjoyment of this space?

- *Noise...hot sun...too much work.*

As with any upscale destination spa, the complete environment – the surround – is planned specifically to nourish all the senses. And so it can be with your home spa.

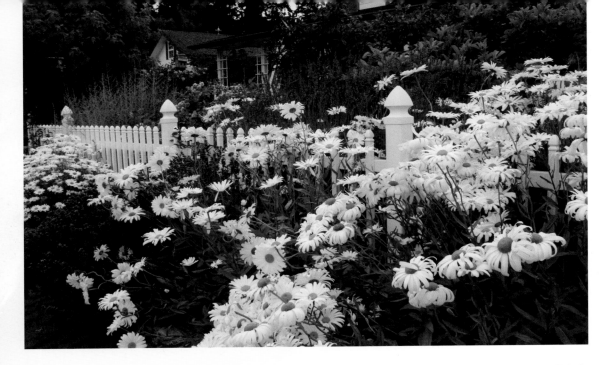

DESIGN ESSENTIALS FOR THE SANCTUARY GARDEN

Plants

The garden needs to be planned to grow herbs for use in your spa remedies, of course, but more than that, you are creating space to experience the hand-blended treatments. This is your outdoor spa. Its space is defined with ornamental plants that are chosen for hedging privacy, overhead natural canopies and living walls.

For an overall calming effect, blend fragrant plants and soothing color palettes. Your plant choices become healers, aromatherapy, and sensory stimulators. Use them to fill in around seating, pathways and other hardscape in the garden. (It goes without saying that you would avoid plants with spiky or thorny habits.)

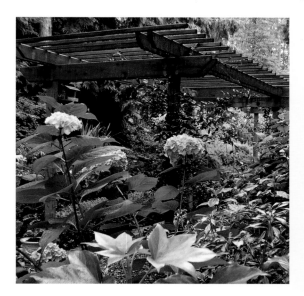

Security

Add structure, like a pergola, or plant trees as an overhead canopy. This provides a sense of shelter and comfort, much like the ceiling of a house. Garden walls, whether living plants or built structures, define the area and make us feel secure and safe.

Privacy

Create a haven. Privacy screens and hedges block out uninvited eyes and undesirable views.

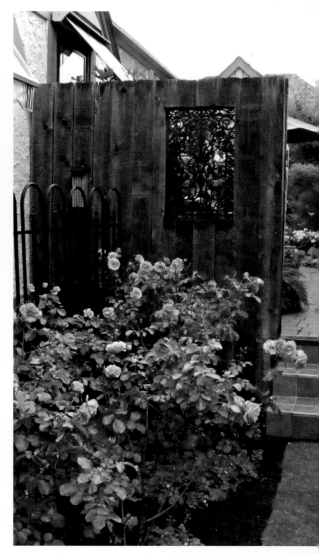

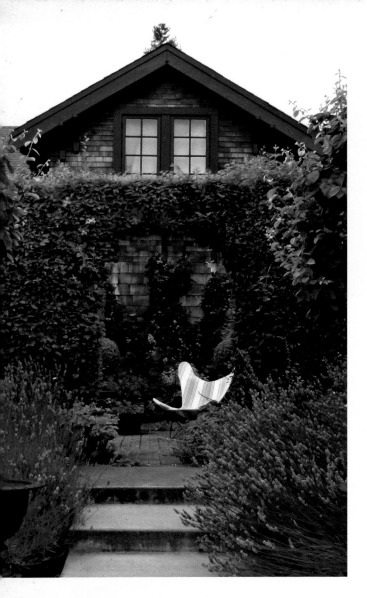

Rooms

Divide an area from the busy activity of an outdoor space. A distinct entry point trough an arbor or gate reinforces the idea that you have walked into a special space.

Outdoor living

Are you planning for an outdoor bed, shower, bathtub, hot tub, or seating? This is where comfort is imperative. Bring all of the luxuries of home outside. Create a sleeping area in a quiet place shaded from bright daylight. For a seating respite, choose comfortable outdoor furniture. Place it where it captures your favorite time of day or where you will frequent it. Buffer a bathtub or shower from prying eyes, inclement weather and intruders by surrounding it with plants and privacy structures. If a hot tub is already installed as part of the home, create a relaxing view by planting a beautiful tree as a focus or bring in elegant, colorful pottery

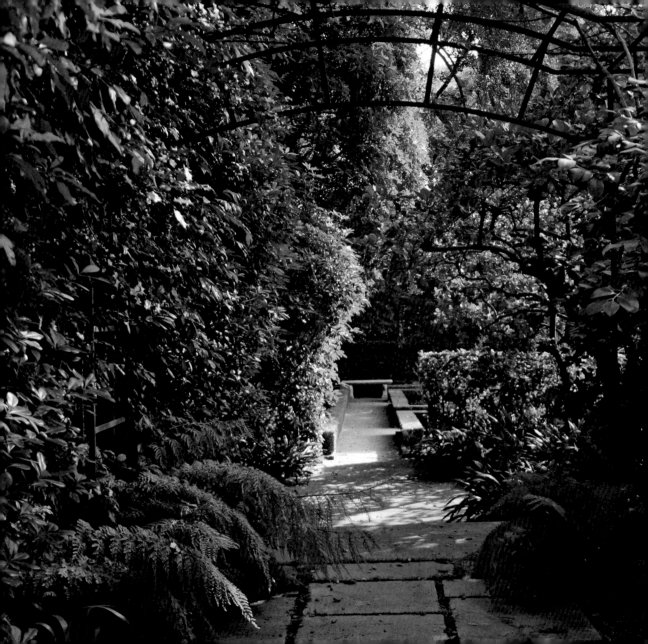

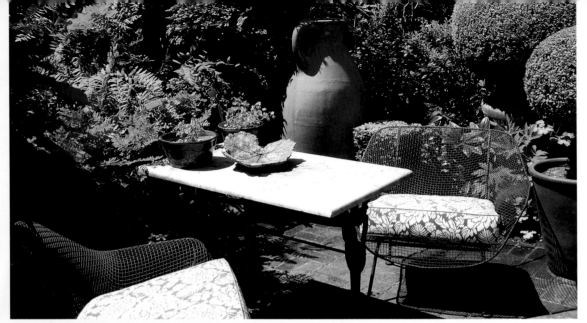

Even the simplicity of a small patio or balcony becomes a retreat by placing pottery and fragrant herbs to create your surroundings. Finish with comfortable, deep-cushioned seating and a table.

and surround it with colorful plants. Look for ways to integrate the hot tub into the landscape so it doesn't stick out like a sore thumb. For the undesirable views you cannot change, hide them with fencing or large plants that billow and camouflage.

Personal space

Be selfish, this is a place to read, eat, sleep, bathe or shower. Make it personal.

Protection from the elements

Know your garden space well by watching how the sun plays in it – note the warmth of the morning sun or a cool shady spot from the heat of the sun. Position your space very purposefully. If your favorite spot needs shade from hot sun, consider a pergola that will filter the light and cool the air. You can create spaces to use year-round by adding a garden shed that can be heated and gives protection from rain and snow. Or re-style a greenhouse once used for nurturing plants into a living space to nurture your soul.

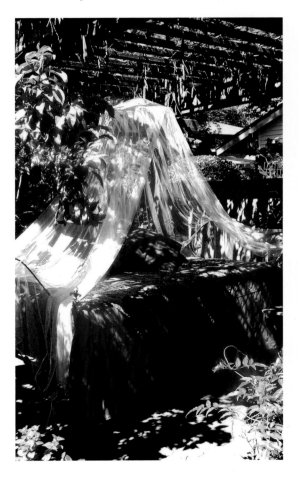

Sound

Outside noise influences our ability to relax and many times in a garden it is sound we cannot control, like a noisy street or neighborhood. You may need to add desirable sounds: water bubbling from a pottery fountain or the splash of a waterfall to help drown out unwelcome noise. Plants can also be strategically placed, such as bamboo and tall ornamental grasses, to catch wind and rustle organic sounds through a space. Use plant varieties to encourage birds to nest and shelter, to add their vocalization as background noise.

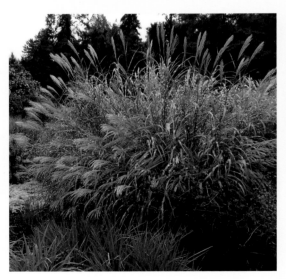

The Importance of Texture

Much has been said about the sense of smell, sight and sound, but the sense of touch brings heightened awareness as well. Soothing massage, water against skin in a bath, the feel of hot or cold temperature; the tingle of skin by application of the spa treatments, everything done by touch. This shows another element to be mindful of in a sanctuary space: the texture and feel of plants, fabrics and furniture.

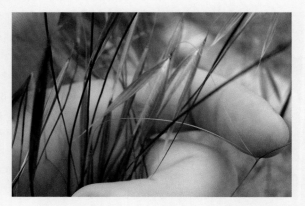

In a garden, plants with plush leaves like lamb's ear (*Stachys byzantina*), the quilted leaves of hosta, and soft ornamental grasses add texture. The bark of trees with peeling layers, like paperbark maple (*Acer griseum*), or the soft, smooth sheen of Tibetan flowering cherry (*Prunus serrula*) are visual texture in mixed plantings. Consider adding touchable flowers and seed heads, like ornamental Alliums, the downy, soft flowers of Spanish lavender (*Lavandula stoechas*) and the silky fragrant petals of gardenia.

Fabrics against skin quicken the sense of touch, but there is a remembrance of how it will feel just by the sight of the texture.

It is not hard for many of us to imagine an early experience of raw, scratchy wool on freshly showered skin. Fabric from linens, towels, robes, pillows and furniture covers needs to feel comforting, embracing. For fabrics that touch skin after a treatment, choose textures of natural, soft cotton, and the smoothness of silk.

If you have the luxury to create a dedicated, private spa space and are able to select the material for construction, give careful thought to the texture of floors and walls. The closer to a natural material such as bamboo or smooth wood, the more comforting the texture and feel of the space.

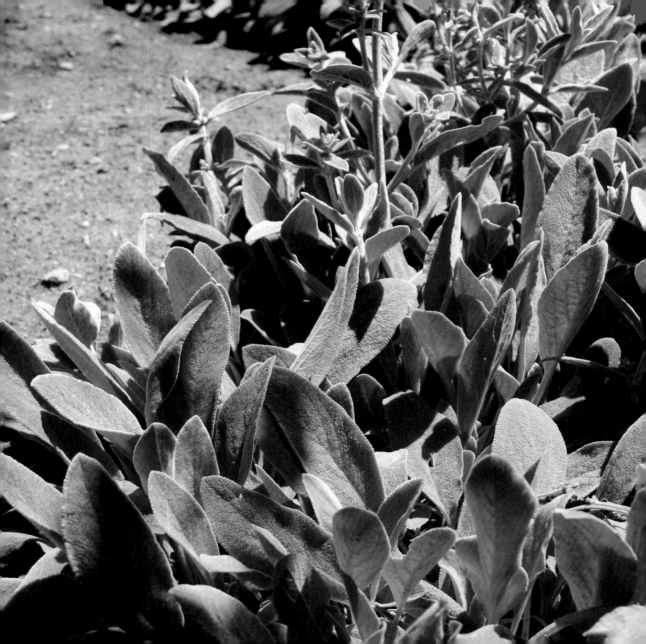

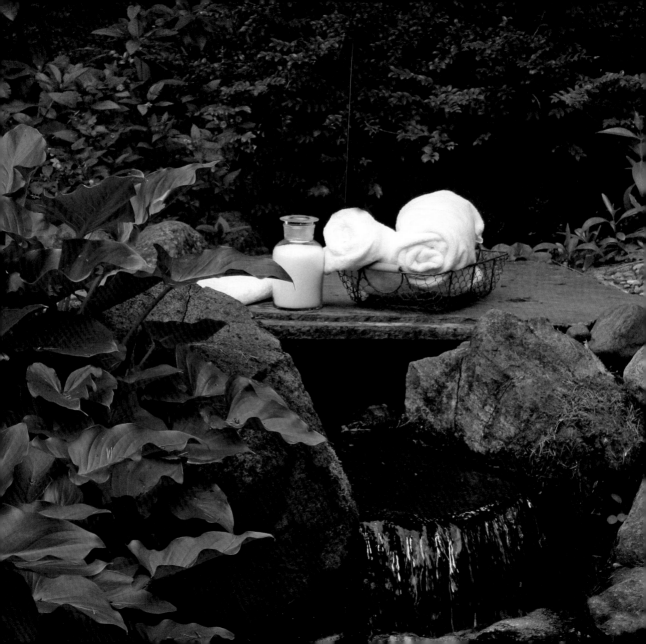

You know the moment you walk through the door of a resort spa. You feel indulged. Natural wood, greenery and earthen tones surround you. The fragrance of fresh herbs lingers in the air. You are handed a fluffy, cotton robe to change in to. The music, the lights, the fragrance, all capture your senses. The atmosphere is intentional and carefully designed to envelope and prepare you for the rest of the treatment. The environment is really a part of the healing. It begins to lower your blood pressure and blot out the stress of the day.

Find your space

Go ahead, steal ideas from luxurious destination spas and recreate the experience at home. Most of us do not have the extravagance of space to set aside as the spa room, so get creative and find ways to make space. Choose a relaxing area where you can feel separate from the usual activity of the home. The bathroom is typically the chosen space because of the access to water and a tub, plus a door that locks! Keep a basket of spa essentials ready for those times you choose to make the everyday bathroom into your own private spa destination. If there is another room inside that is more relaxing, then use it. Not all spa treatments need a tub.

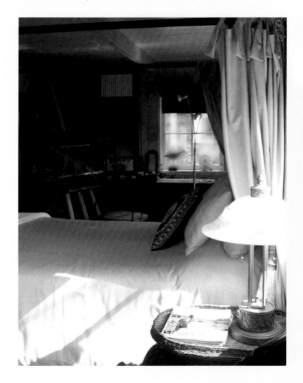

CREATE THE ATMOSPHERE

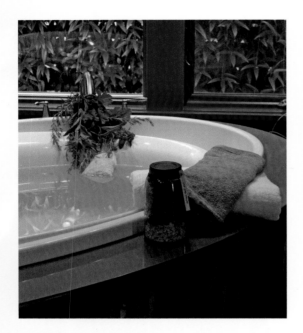

Sound

Soft music or the sounds of birds and nature are good for relaxation during soaking times. Create a playlist that is used just for spa time. Music is a memory trigger and targeting the right kind of music or sounds to your spa time will encourage calm and relaxation. Or, if you're in a playful mood, step up the music beat to go with invigorating scrubs or foot treatments. Nature sounds take away the artificial buzz that music can be; the sound of waves crashing on the beach, birds and even the gentle drum of rain clears your mind. You can design the mood with sound.

Lighting

Lighting that can be adjusted from bright to dim is helpful. Add a lamp that uses a 3-way bulb or replace the regular light switch in the room with a dimmer switch. Bright light is needed for scrubs and treatments. But you'll want to dim the lights or use candles when using relaxation soaks, steams or massage.

Color

Color is an important mood maker. Greens and natural earth tones hues are the most relaxing. No need to paint all the walls with color in an existing space, but introduce calming, cool colors with pillows, linens and towels.

Color in a Sanctuary Space

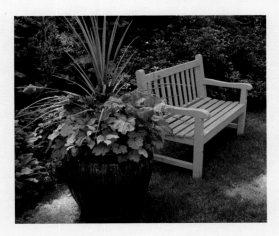

Inside the home or out in the garden, what the eyes sees affects emotion. Color is an important part of setting a mood. A few general guidelines:

- Warm colors – like reds, oranges and yellows – are for spaces with activity. They are the colors of fire and heat, and tend to make a space feel degrees warmer than it actually is. For a more relaxing experience, avoid true reds, which are known to increase blood pressure and heart rate. It is much more soothing to bring in paler pinks and peach – warm colors, but not so strong.

- Cool colors, like shades of blue, calm and lower blood pressure.
- Hues of green make a space feel degrees cooler.
- Jewel tone colors, like deep violets and burgundy, add a luxurious appeal.
- If your space has strong, stark colors, bring in some grey, white or black accents to help blend and play down the dominant tones.
- Neutral colors on walls and floors provide a backdrop for light to bounce off, and invite experimenting with brighter-hued accessories.
- The presence of natural wood, whether in garden fixtures, furniture or floors, suggests calm, whereas painted wood will create a different mood, according to the color you use.

No need to be boring or overwhelming. Well thought out touches of color, outdoors and indoors, like garden pottery, furniture coverings and toss pillows on the bed might just be the simple change you need to enhance your surroundings. You'll know when you've achieved a feeling of sanctuary.

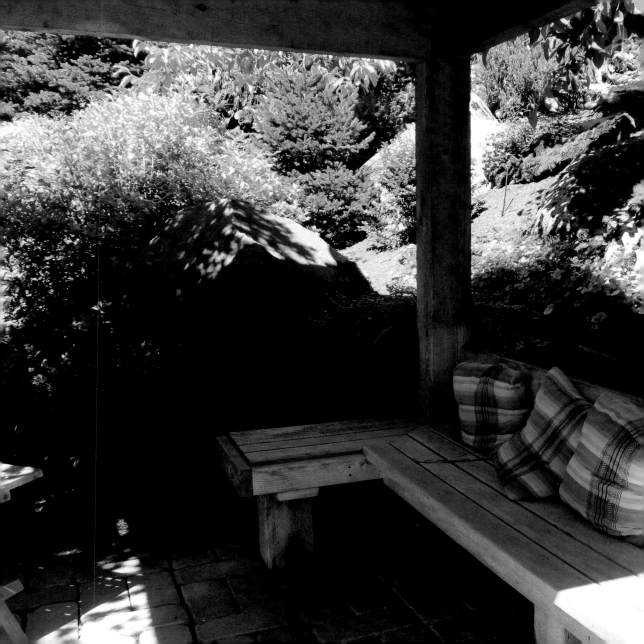

A spa session is your intermission from a busy world. Power down the phone and computer. Your spa time is not intended to be interaction with social media, it is time to pamper yourself.

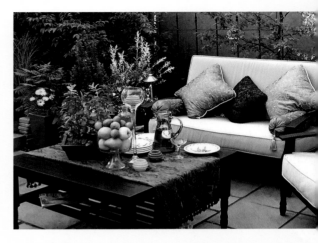

- ***Make space!*** Create a relaxing, healing space in your own home or garden.

- ***Make time!*** Make an appointment with yourself. At the end of a stressful day, steep in a bath of aromatic herbs, to not only clean the daily grime off skin, but allow your mind to let go of things that cannot be taken care of in the moment. Think ahead of a busy time and have a pro-active spa moment. If there is an upcoming event that will be stressful, plan an uplifting sugar body scrub before the event.

- ***Share!*** Welcome friends for a meal, conversation or gathering into the garden. The enchantment of fragrant herbs and peaceful space will soon begin to weave its spell. Strew rosemary and lavender cuttings on pathways and patios to release natural air fresheners when walked upon. Provide rosewater with fresh cut lemon slices for hand washing before and after a meal. Invite girlfriends (or boyfriends) for a foot scrub party. Treat someone special to a private herbal massage or shared bathing.

With those lovely images in our minds, let's turn our attention to the herbs and discover who they are and what they can do to make our lives – and our spa time – delightful.

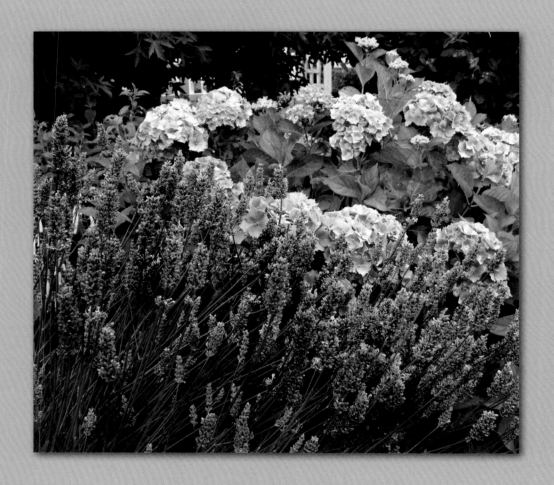

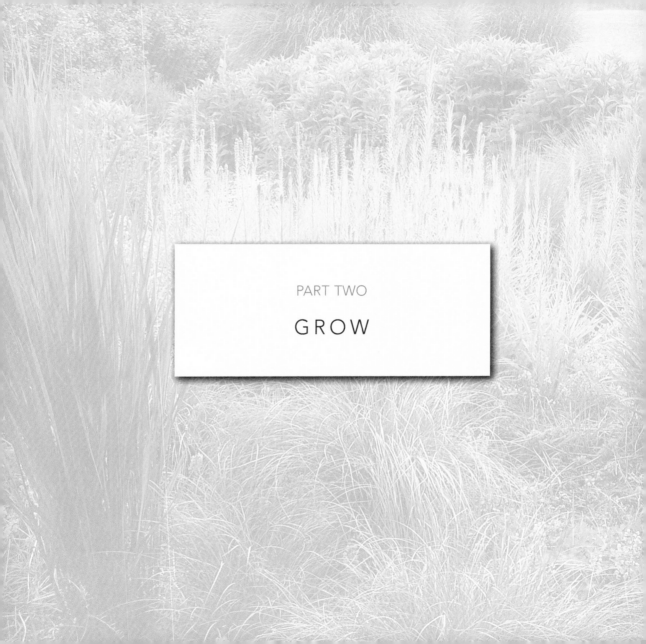

PART TWO

GROW

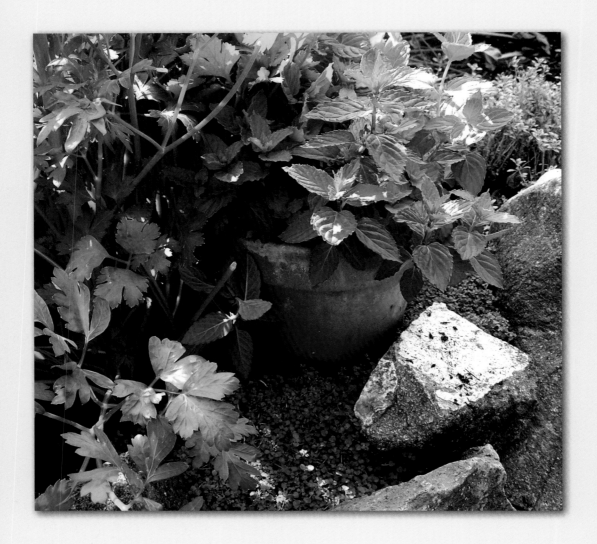

A garden of herbs

becomes a new adventure when you

discover the many ways to use them.

From cooking to crafting, the diversity of flavor and fragrance is the true allure of growing an abundant garden of herbs.

You may already be growing some herbs, whether for their culinary use or their beauty, or both. It might surprise you to know what else they can do for you. Their special qualities can be antiseptic, aromatic, healing, soothing, cooling, stimulating; and you can use the flowers, leaves, stems, oils or roots. In this part of our book, you'll learn about your old favorites and perhaps meet new ones. And then later on, I'll show you what other ingredients are needed to bring a plant into a form that your body can easily utilize – and luxuriate in.

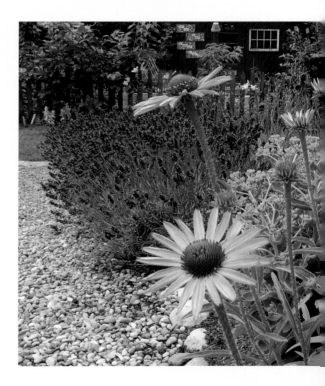

■ ■ ■

What, Exactly, is an Herb?

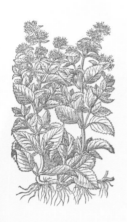

Herbs have captivated gardeners for thousands of years. They inspire us with all they give us. Plants commonly referred to as herbs are familiar culinary varieties such as chives, oregano, and basil, but we hear less about nontraditional plants classified as herbs, such as agave, with leaf sap that can be used to treat burns. Naturopaths and herbal healers may have hundreds of plants they consider herbs, while home gardeners may have only a dozen plants they call herbs. Thinking from this perspective, herbs can be identified culturally as well as botanically. Even if you have not read a single herb garden book, chances are you recognize herbs by how they permeate legends, literature and lyrics – and the way we use them to enhance our lifestyle.

More than ten thousand books have been written about herbs over the centuries, yet we still may wonder what really classifies a plant as an herb. The first entry in the American Heritage Dictionary states that the origin of the word herb is Middle English, via old French, from the Latin herba. It is defined as "any plant with leaves, seeds or flowers used for flavoring food, medicine or perfume." The second entry definition has a botanical bias: "any seed-bearing plant that does not have a woody stem and dies to the ground after flowering." Just reading these two definitions encompasses numerous plants and explains why so many people are confused about what, exactly, constitutes the group of plants called herbs.

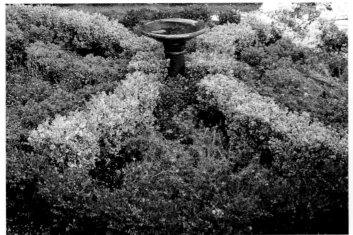

information was vital to the types of plants harvested for a specific purpose such as healing, food preparation, and perfume. Use of the word herb evolved to mean plants that had a specific use or purpose because of an active ingredient. Trees and shrubs can fit this definition if they have a useful purpose, such as the woody shrub witch hazel, widely known for its astringent qualities.

In the earliest beginnings of man, plants were harvested from the wild for many uses, then gardened for their prized value. Historically, plants were classified in three basic categories: trees, shrubs, and herbs. If it was not a tree or a shrub, it was an herb. In other words, herbs were plants that lacked a "permanent" woody stem or structure. However, in the warmer USDA climate zones 8 and above, some herbs do not die back to the ground in winter. In addition, herbs can be annual, biennial, or perennial, breaking down the notion that herbs are only perennial and herbaceous. As plant knowledge expanded, accurate

Botanists and horticulturalists can find middle ground by defining an herb as any type of plant cultivated for its usefulness in flavoring, perfume, or for cosmetic and medicinal uses.

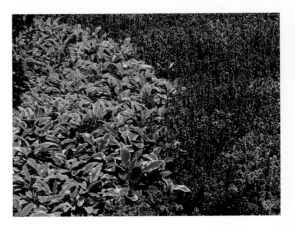

How's your Latin? Botanical Latin names can be vexing and intimidating. Sometimes Latin pronunciation rolls off the tongue, but more often than not, the words stumble out uncomfortably. Rather than be uncomfortable with botanical Latin, learn to embrace why we need to know it. The use and knowledge of botanical Latin

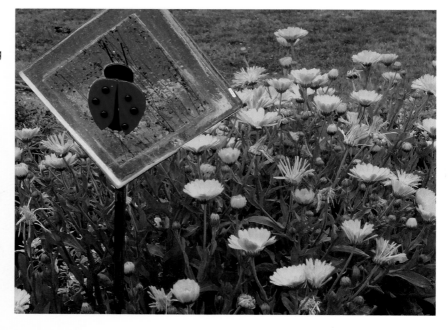

names allows opportunity for gardeners to learn more about an herb, its history and its cultivation. The history of plants can be very revealing about what we need to know to grow them.

Why it matters that we get to know a botanical name

In herb lore and gardening, common names are used more frequently than the proper botanical Latin names. Basil, for instance, is usually listed by its common name rather than the botanical name *Ocimum basilicum*. It has become typical in herb garden writing and on seed packets to use the common name. Most people would not recognize the plant *Petroselinum crispum* unless we also hear its common name, parsley.

Common names of herbs can be a fascinating study all on their own. Common names were given typically because of a plant's appearance or its original use. Consider the name of the herb known as bible leaf or costmary, *Tanacetum balsamita*, named for the lore that a fresh leaf was tucked into bibles for a snack to alleviate hunger during long sermons.

A pitfall of common names is that they can vary by geographic location, which makes plant identification confusing. Knowing the botanical name is vital when we're using herbs for consumption, whether internal or external. Much misunderstanding and even trouble can come from relying solely on common names.

An example of name confusion is pot marigold, which is botanically *Calendula officinalis*. The name "marigold" conjures up the image of the familiar golden orange flower *Tagetes patula*, used as a summer annual in most gardens. But these are two very different plants, pot marigold (*Calendula*) is revered for its gentle, healing qualities in skin preparations, while the common marigold, *Tagetes patula*, is better known for repelling bugs in the garden. Getting the two confused without proper botanical identification could result in a

serious skin rash if the wrong variety were used in a cosmetic preparation.

Officinalis or Officinale?

When we look at the terminology of botanical language we can discover clues to the ways herbs were used in the daily lives of our ancestors. The specific label *officinalis* or *officinale*, meaning "of the druggist's storeroom," signifies that in past recorded history the plant was used commercially as medicine. In the eighteen century, as Swedish botanist Carl Linnaeus was bestowing names on plants, many herbs were already common and familiar to herbalists. Linnaeus had to decide between a plant's official status to identify it or another descriptive word for the species – and so *officinalis* was tagged onto an herb that was being regularly used for medicine at the time. It gives us a much deeper sense of history when we encounter ordinary garden herbs with the species name "*officinalis.*"

HERBS FOR SKIN CARE: NATURAL VS. "NATURAL"

Cosmetic use of plant material is rooted deep in our collective past, with records and recipes handed down through the ages. The awareness of plant material used as healing and aromatic skin preparations

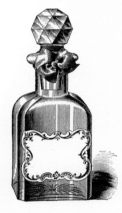

has been with us since biblical times. And then came Theron T. Pond, a New Yorker who learned about a wonderful herb that the local Native Americans were using as a topical application for the skin. In 1846, Pond mixed a simple blend of witch hazel, oil, wax and water that was developed as "Pond's Extract." This was the early beginnings of what is now a multi-billion-dollar cosmetic industry.

The latest trend in commercial skin products is to use "natural" materials in blends of shampoos and lotions. But if you look at the ingredients list of a bottle that shows an herb on its label and makes a point of its herbal lineage, you will often discover that there is little or none of that herb within. Why would that be? Synthetics are cheaper, easier to mass produce, and they avoid the process of growing and harvesting. Most skin care products require a shelf life as well as consistency in color and texture. It is all those long-lettered mystery words in the ingredient list that give them those qualities. The product has to look and smell good and be able to be shipped in hot and cold weather all over the world.

Missing or lost in the long list of ingredients is the pure essence of the plants, which gives potions their true effectiveness. This is where an herbal spa garden becomes your provider. Using the freshness of the garden, you are the alchemist that preserves and infuses all of the properties that indulge the skin and senses.

You, the alchemist. For many of us, the idea of using our own herbs in skin care recipes is very intriguing, but it tends to be lost in the notion that it can be

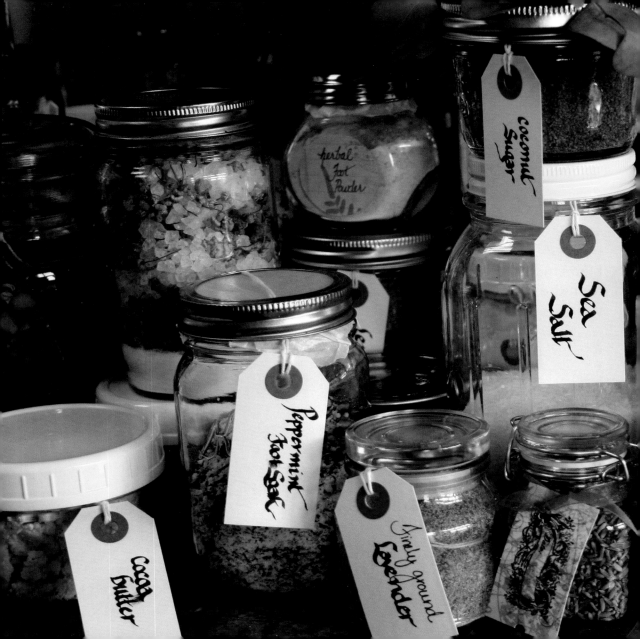

complicated – too much work. It conjures up the image of a dungeon of boiling beakers with steam rising into the air… or needing to know scientific substances and how to pronounce words like isopropyl myristate. The real discovery – after a bit of learning about herbal plant qualities and ingredients used for skin and spa treatments – is that it is all really basic and easy to do. Most of the makings can be found in the kitchen and the garden.

Homemade preparations direct from the garden

To know what to grow and what type of recipes to use them in, it begins with learning about the herb plants and their properties – which ones are antiseptic, aromatic, healing, soothing, cooling, stimulating. And then knowing what part of the plant is to be used: the flower, leaves, stems, oils or roots. Once you've become familiar with the assets of the herbs, then you'll want to learn what ingredients are needed to get a plant into a useable from – making it spread-able, spray-able and into a form that the body can easily utilize.

Fresh, handmade recipes have a different look and feel than what is found on the drugstore shelf, because the major components rely on all the wonderful qualities of the plants. By making homemade preparations you are the quality control expert and can be picky with the ingredients that are used in the recipes. You have control over freshness and purity and can choose the ingredients to avoid allergies or skin sensitivities. Your preparations allow more of the healing properties to go directly where they are needed.

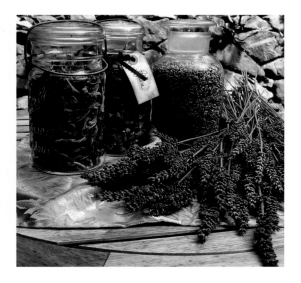

Sourcing Your Herb Plants

In selecting your herb plants, you want to be sure they have been grown organically. No chemical residues wanted! Buy local from farmers markets and garden shops. Most growers at local markets are happy to tell you how they raised and cared for their plants. In nurseries and garden shops, there are not typically signs or labels to say how the herb plants were grown before they got to the nursery. Ask the staff if the herbs were grown organically. If they are not grown organically or you are not sure, don't worry: you can typically grow perennial herbs in your garden and just not use them cosmetically the first year. Let them go through a season of dying back. The new growth will be the way you grow them – naturally and by organic methods! After a full year cycle, the residual of past chemical use should be leached out and gone. If you're planting

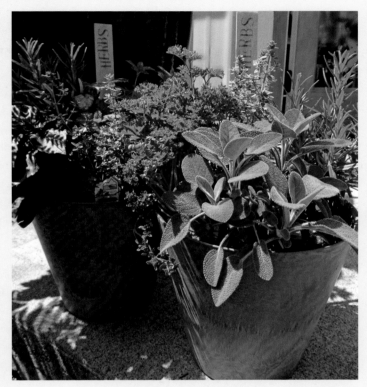

from seed, seeds will be labeled organic on the packets, but it is truly how the plants are grown that will make them safe to use for cosmetics.

Sourcing Herbs and Supplies Beyond the Garden

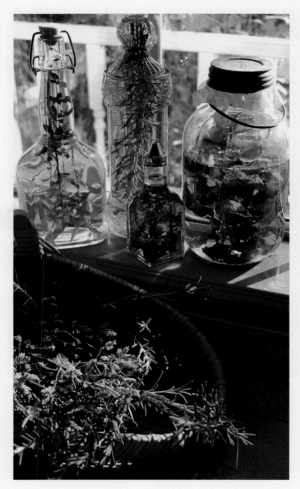

Not every garden will have what is needed in a recipe at the same time. Some things you simply cannot grow or have enough of and you need to source them. Shop at local herb farms, food co-ops, farmer's markets, and health food stores. Online resources are abundant and offer just about anything needed to create your spa products, including dried herbs, base ingredients and packaging supplies. Always source from reputable, trusted companies (see Resources for a listing of some I use.) There is not much in the way of regulation for quality with dried herbs and essential oils, so do some homework, read their catalog and ask about their products. Suppliers who specialize in herbs for food and cosmetic purposes, and companies who supply massage and natural health practitioners, are good places to start. I have found good resources are transparent about their products and won't hide behind a fancy label; they tell you where it came from and what is in it.

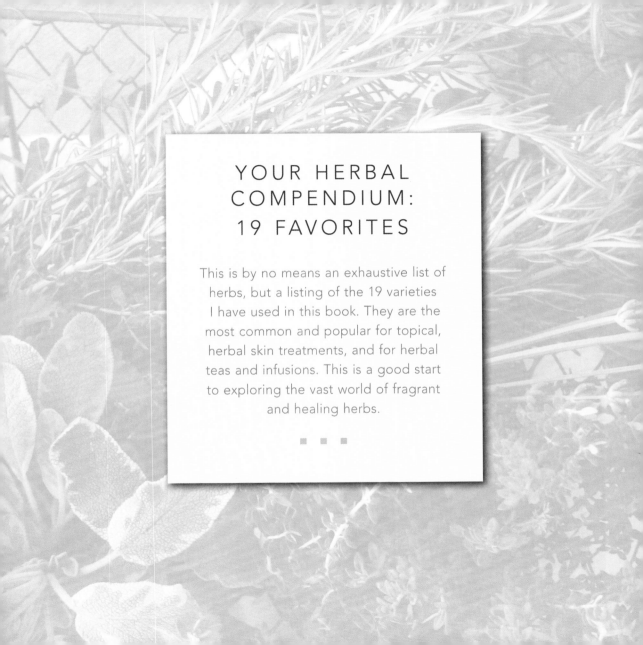

YOUR HERBAL COMPENDIUM: 19 FAVORITES

This is by no means an exhaustive list of herbs, but a listing of the 19 varieties I have used in this book. They are the most common and popular for topical, herbal skin treatments, and for herbal teas and infusions. This is a good start to exploring the vast world of fragrant and healing herbs.

■ ■ ■

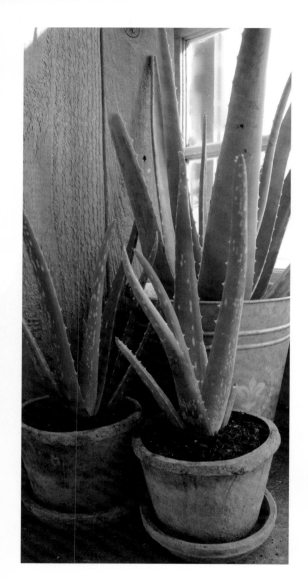

Aloe Vera

Common name: Aloe Vera

Botanical Name: *Aloe vera*

Culture: USDA Zones 9 to 11. Protect from frost. Grow indoors in bright light. Commonly grown as a houseplant.

Properties: Skin healing and repair.

Parts Used: Fresh sap inside the leaf.

Notes: Split the leaf lengthwise and open to reveal the clear gel inside. The sap in the leaves is soothing and healing. Its finest reputation is for the treatment of burns. It's well worth growing a pot of aloe vera as a houseplant to keep a constant supply of fresh leaves for first aid.

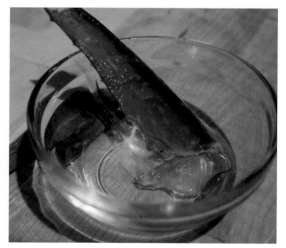

■ Basil

Common Name: Basil

Botanical Name: *Ocimum basilicum*

Culture: Annual. Leafy bushy plants tender to frost. Needs full sun and rich, well-drained soil. Pinch off the flowers through the growing season to encourage bushy growth.

Properties: Uplifting, energizing, anti-depressant.

Parts Used: Leaves, best when used fresh. Can be frozen or dried, but the fragrance and flavor will diminish when dried.

Notes: This is the classic culinary type of basil. Popular in pesto and Italian dishes, use the true Italian basils for their strong fragrant notes of camphor and clove. Look for the varieties 'Genovese' and 'Napoletano'. The rich burgundy leaves of 'Red Rubin' or 'Osmin' will infuse a natural rosy color into skin care products.

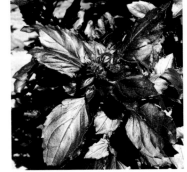

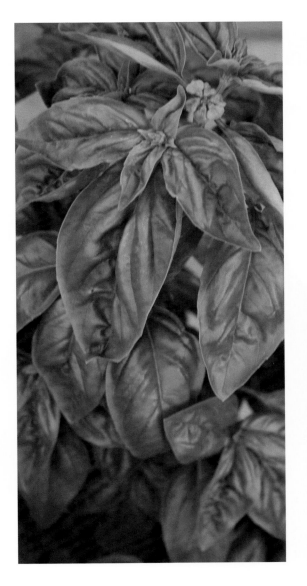

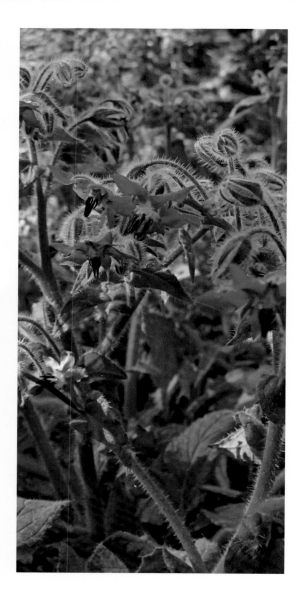

■ Borage

Common Name: Borage

Botanical Name: *Borago officinalis*

Culture: Annual. Grows up to 36 inches tall. Easy to start from seed and self-sows readily if the seed heads remain on the plants at the end of the season.

Properties: Healing, uplifting, refreshing.

Parts used: Flower petals and leaves. Pick fresh flowers, just as they become fully open. Cut and use fresh leaves in season; they will not store or dry well.

Notes: Known as the herb of gladness for its positive effect on mood. The rough textured leaves are full of vitamins and minerals and can be eaten fresh in salad. The flowers infused in water are a delicate tonic wash for sensitive and dry skin. The light blue petals have pleasant cucumber-like aroma, good for summertime beverages and herbal ice cubes, too.

▪Calendula

Common Name: Calendula, pot marigold

Botanical Name: *Calendula officinalis*

Culture: Annual. Full sun to part shade. Easy to grow and start from seed. Grows 1 to 2 feet tall. Deadhead faded blooms to encourage repeat blooming.

Properties: Soothing, astringent and cleansing.

Parts used: Flower petals, use fresh or dried.

Notes: "Pot marigold" should not to be confused with the garden-type marigold *(Tagetes)*. Use the flower heads and petals of Calendula fresh and dried to heal irritated and rashy skin. It is very gentle and soothing to all skin types. An invaluable herb infused in salves for first-aid preparations. The deep golden-orange petals add natural color to lotions and ointments.

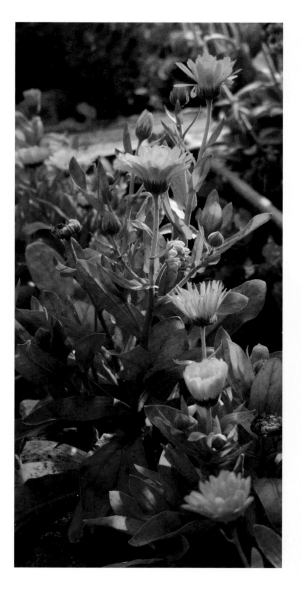

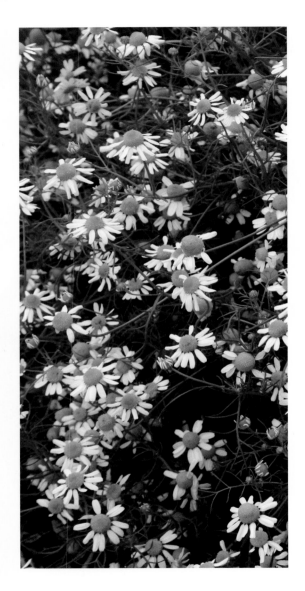

■ Chamomile

Common Name: Chamomile, ground apple, lawn chamomile

Botanical Name: *Chamaemelum nobile; Matricaria recutita*

Culture: USDA Zone 4. German chamomile (*Matricaria recutita*) is a tall-growing annual that heavily re-seeds if allowed. Roman chamomile (*Chamemelum nobile*) is a low-growing carpet-like perennial. Grows up to 12 inches tall and spreads by creeping rhizomes. Full sun to part shade. Best in well-draining soil. Both chamomile flowers look similar and are used interchangeably in cosmetics; Roman chamomile will have a stronger fragrance. Grow the variety 'Bodegold' (*Matricaria recutita* 'Bodegold') for its high essential oil quality.

Properties: Soothing, cleansing, emollient, reduces puffiness.

Parts Used: Flowers, use fresh and dried.

Notes: The word chamomile originates from Greek, meaning earth apple or "apple on the ground," referring to its sweet apple fragrance. The flowers are very mild and gentle, healing to skin. Good for use in hair rinses, skin lotions and balms and bath blends. Tea made from the flowers is well known as a calming bedtime drink and can be soothing to an upset tummy.

Planting a Chamomile Lawn

Roman chamomile (*Chamaemelum nobile*) is the traditional variety used for lawns and can be mowed just like common turf grass. It is fragrant and soft underfoot, perfect for a outdoor path or sitting area in a spa garden. The more it is walked upon, the better it will thicken and form a dense mat.

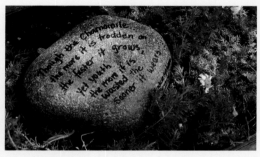

"For though the camomile, the more it is trodden on, the faster it grows, so youth, the more it is wasted, the sooner it wears."
William Shakespeare, Henry IV, Part 1

To design an herbal lawn into a garden, start small. Establishing an herbal lawn is very different from establishing traditional grass. The beginning stages of growth and filling in take diligent weeding and care. A large herbal lawn is costly to plant, but small areas (under one hundred square feet) and green pathways are very elegant and effective when planted in ground-hugging herbs. Once established, it will evolve to lower maintenance as the creeping plants knit together and form a thick carpet.

Take time to prepare the ground before planting. Weed thoroughly and clean out rocks and debris. Add 3 to 4 inches of weed-free organic compost and turn into the soil. If the area is hard clay-type soil in the sun, loosen and add sandy compost mix to encourage good drainage. Rake, smooth and level. A good rule of thumb is to plant an established 4-inch plant; 4 plants per square foot. The goal is to have plants knit together quickly to establish solid coverage. As an alternative, seed can be broadcast over the prepared ground. Cover with a thin layer of soil and keep moist. Try to establish plants or seeds in cooler parts of the year when there is better moisture in the soil. Keep pets and heavy foot traffic off the area and be very meticulous about weeding for the first few seasons. The seeds will not take competition well while trying to establish.

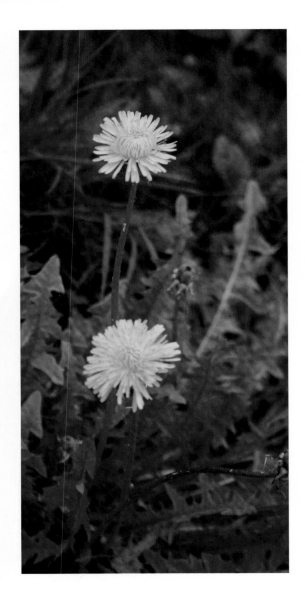

■ Dandelion

Common Name: Dandelion

Botanical Name: *Taraxacum officinale*

Culture: Annual. Yes, this is THAT common weed. Not readily planted in most gardens, it just shows up and sows freely in open areas of lawn. Grows up to 12 inches with a bright yellow flower.

Properties: Cleansing, tonic.

Parts Used: Leaves and flowers. Use fresh in season, it does not dry well. Harvest flowers just as they fully open.

Notes: This lowly weed is actually a highly regarded herb and as early as the 16th century was established as an official drug. The leaves are high in vitamins and can be eaten raw in salads. The leaves infused in water are a nourishing, cleansing tonic for facial steams and moisturizing bath blends. A water made with the bright flowers make a simple and effective face wash. The root dried, roasted and ground is a classic coffee substitute. The root will also yield a deep magenta dye to color lotions and massage oils. All parts of dandelion are best used fresh and make the perfect addition to a healing springtime spa treatment.

■ Eucalyptus

Common Name: Eucalyptus, gum tree, snow gum

Botanical Name: *Eucalyptus* spp.

Culture: USDA Zone 8. Tree. Needs full sun and gritty, well-draining soil. Plant in areas where it has the most sun and warmth. If hit by frost, the leaves will die but typically will regrow from the roots.

Properties: Antiseptic, antifungal, healing, stimulating

Parts used: Leaf, fresh and dried.

Notes: The volatile greenish oil extracted from the leaves of eucalyptus is well-documented and studied as effective antiseptic and deodorant. The strong camphor fragrance and healing properties are favored in chest congestion and cough preparations. As a spa treatment, the cleansing qualities are used to add aroma to steams and sauna to stimulate the pores of the skin.

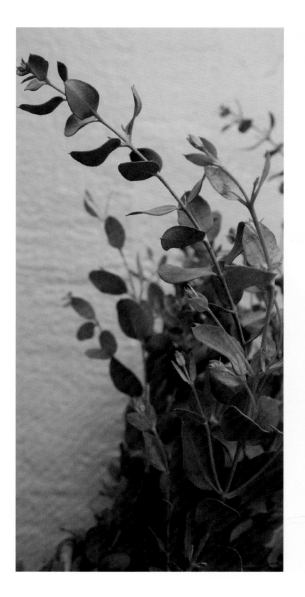

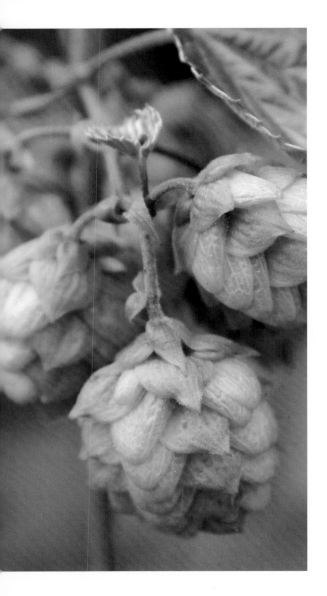

■ Hops

Common Name: Hops, common hop, bine

Botanical Name: *Humulus lupulus*

Culture: USDA Zone 3. Herbaceous vine grows 15 to 25 feet. Full sun with well-draining soil. Easy to grow, very fast growing and vigorous. The plant will die to the ground after a first frost in the fall, the vines can be removed every winter and new shoots will emerge in the spring.

Properties: Sedative, sleep inducing.

Parts Used: Flowers. Pick the flowers when they are fully open and ripe. The dried flowers need to be used within a few months of harvest or the fragrance will become unpleasant.

Notes: Known for their narcotic effect, hops are used in relaxation and sleep inducing mixes. This is the same flower that is used in beer making. The flower is a small yellowish bloom that ripens into papery bracts called strobiles, which contain glands filled with a powdery substance; it's that substance, containing bitter tonic chemicals, that gives its distinctive aroma. Hops have a long and interesting medicinal history, some of which is described in Margaret Grieve's classic 1931 compilation, *A Modern Herbal*. One recipe for a topical hop salve is to be used as a "fomentation for swelling of a painful nature, inflammation and rheumatic pains."

■ Lavender

Common Name: Lavender

Botanical Name: *Lavandula*

Culture: USDA Zone 5. Herbaceous to semi-evergreen perennial. Varieties grow from 12 inches to 4 feet tall. Full sun. Prefers dry, rocky soil and dislikes too much compost or richness. Must have well-draining soil to prevent the roots from rotting and brown-rotting at the base of the plant. Use English varieties such as 'Munstead' or 'Hidcote' for a sweet fragrance, or the hybrid cross intermedias such as 'Grosso' and 'Provence' for heavy flower and oil production.

Properties: Astringent, stimulating, cleansing, healing.

Parts Used: Flower buds. Use fresh and dried.

Notes: Known for its classic old-fashioned fragrance; a very soothing, healing herb. The essential oil is readily available and one of the few essential oils gentle enough to use directly on skin (individuals should test for skin sensitivity before use). Good for burns, skin irritations, oily skin and blemishes. Different types of lavender produce oils that have higher levels of camphor, making them good for cleansing and antibacterial properties. Lavender can be used in many diverse ways including spray mists, teas, lotions and balms, bath blends and sachets.

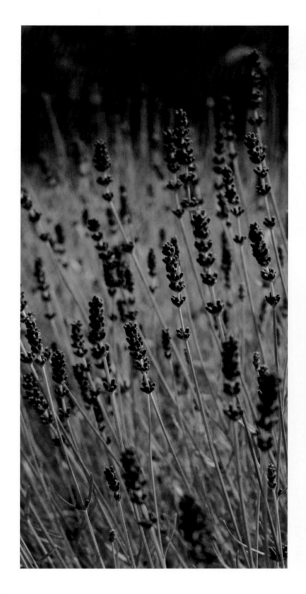

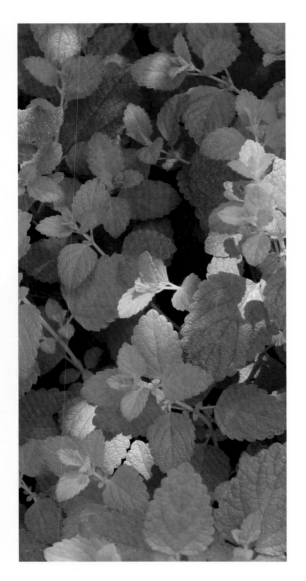

■ Lemon Balm

Common Name: Lemon Balm

Botanical Name: *Melissa officinalis*

Culture: USDA Zone 3. Aggressive spreading perennial. Height up to 2 feet. Easy to grow in average soil

Properties: Cleansing, antiseptic, warming.

Parts Used: Leaves, use fresh and dried

Notes: In medieval times, lemon balm was prescribed for numerous ailments such as a cure for toothache, mad dog bites, skin sores, and as a tonic for melancholy. Lemon balm is the main ingredient of "Carmelite water," a brew of lemon balm leaves, other spices and herbs in alcohol used as an eau de toilette. In the garden, the leaves have a fresh aroma of soapy lemons when rubbed or crushed. Pick leaves through the summer for fresh recipes. Good for astringent herbal waters, warming baths and facials.

Lemon Verbena

Common Name: Lemon verbena

Botanical Name: *Aloysia triphylla*

Culture: USDA Zone 8. Prefers rich soil in full sun. A deciduous woody shrub up to 10 feet tall in climates where it is hardy. In USDA zone 7 or under, grow as a tender (not hardy to frost) perennial. Will reach up to 5 feet, but needs to be protected from hard frost. The roots may survive down to 20 degrees F. if mulched and protected. In cold winter areas, plant in container gardens and bring indoors for the winter.

Properties: Astringent, healing

Parts Used: Leaves, use fresh and dried.

Notes: This is a must addition to the herb garden, even where it is not hardy outside. It grows fast in the heat of the summer, you can then harvest all the leaves before the first frost. The leaves emit a wonderful lemon-drop fragrance when they are rubbed and crushed. The dried leaves will hold their fragrance in the drying process. Soothing spa lotions, bath blends and salves will have a subtle lemon aroma. Lemon verbena is also a popular and useful addition to sleep pillows and sachets. Oil distilled from the leaves is highly regarded in the perfume and soap industry.

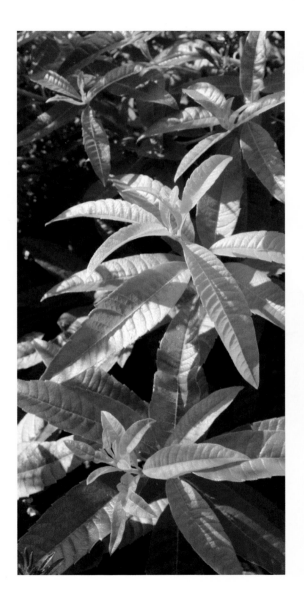

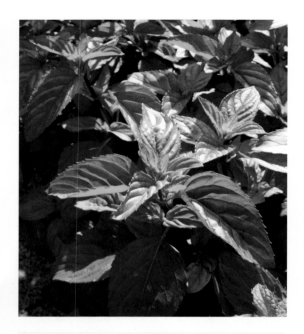

Mint

Common Name: Mint

Botanical Name: *Mentha* spp.

Culture: USDA Zone 4. Herbaceous, aggressive, spreading perennial. Grows up to 2 feet tall. Likes rich, moist soil in full sun. For cosmetic use and teas, grow spearmint *(Mentha spicata)* and true peppermint *(Mentha x piperita piperita)*.

Properties: Stimulating, cleansing.

Parts Used: Leaves, use fresh and dried

Notes: A classic aromatic herb that is healing and astringent. Very refreshing for use in skin lotions, foot soaks, spray mists and bath blends. There are numerous varieties of mints. For a sweeter fragrance and flavor use spearmint. For rich, healing qualities use true peppermint.

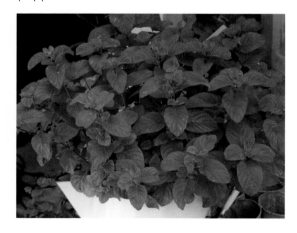

A Quick Chronicle on Mint

Mint is referenced in the Bible and in Greek and Roman writings. Remnants of mint have been found in Egyptian tombs dating back to 1000 B.C. A Greek myth tells us a story of seduction and jealousy. It concerns the nymph Minthe, who was caught in the arms of the husband of Queen Persephone. The queen in a jealous rage is said to have metamorphosed Minthe into a pungent plant to be trampled on.

▪ Parsley

Common Name: Parsley, garden parsley

Botanical Name: *Petroselinum crispum*

Culture: USDA Zone 4. Biennial. Typically grown as an annual. Likes full sun and well-draining soil.

Properties: calming, refreshing; rich source of vitamins.

Parts Used: Leaves, best when used fresh, can be dried.

Notes: The curly variety and flat leaf Italian variety can be used interchangeably. The fresh leaves can be chewed as a breath freshener. Tinctures, salves and infusions made with parley are all very healing to problem skin. Use as a gentle face and body wash to help heal acne and eczema.

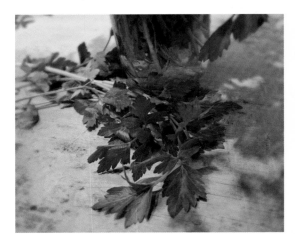

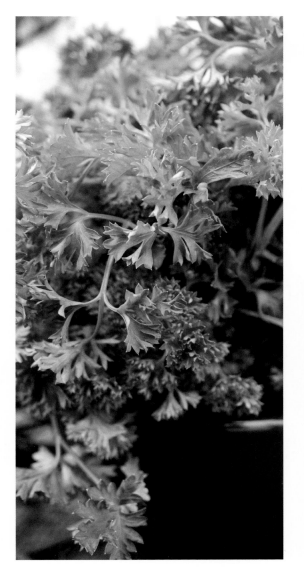

Did you know?
Parsley: a garnish of many virtues

Most people are familiar with parsley as the small scrap of green leaf that sits on the dinner plate at a restaurant. Or maybe the first herb in a '70s song refrain. It has become so commonplace that we hardly notice it there anymore, thus reducing parsley to a scraping after a meal. What relegated it to the side of a plate in the first place? Parsley (*Petroselinum crispum*) in Greek history was one of the most revered herbs, highly esteemed and used in victors' crowns in games; parsley wreaths adorned tombs to show respect for the dead. Greek gardens were bordered with parsley and rue. The medicinal qualities take up pages of old herbals: cleansing, healing, odor neutralizing, a poultice of leaves said to remedy bites and stings – the list goes on. Its virtues extend from the roots to the seed (the seed's volatile oils are extracted for healing purposes). Prominent on this long list of attributes is its ability to overcome strong scents, including garlic. It eases digestion when eaten after a meal, is a breath freshener and is high in minerals and vitamins. So why did parsley become a garnish? Was it meant as an after-meal breath freshener, for color against prepared food – as a signature of an egotistical French chef? Who knows, but the depth of its true herbal attributes contradicts its humble placement on a plate.

▪ Rose

Common Name: Rose

Botanical Name: *Rosa* spp.

Culture: USDA Zones 2 to 7. Shrub. Needs sun, rich soil and good drainage. Height 4 to 6 feet. Best old rose varieties for fragrance: *Rosa* 'Frau Dagmar Hastrup', *Rosa rugosa* 'Hansa', *Rosa* 'Rose du Roi', damask rose *(Rosa damascena)* varieties, 'Madame Hardy' or 'Rose de Rescht', 'Apothecary's Rose' *(Rosa gallica* 'Officinalis'), Rosa Mundi *(Rosa gallica* 'Versicolor').

Properties: Humectant, cleansing, aromatic.

Parts used: Flower petals, rose hips; fresh and dried.

Notes: Choose highly fragrant, multi-petaled roses and roses that produce good hips. The more fragrant the petals the more essential oil is present. 'Apothecary's Rose' is the traditional variety used for cosmetics and medicine. It is one of the oldest roses in cultivation, with recorded history since 1300 A.D. Historic medicals tout rosewater as being prescribed for many ailments including "purification of the mind." Use fresh, organically grown rose petals in bath blends, spray mists, lotions and balms. Excellent for oily skin to cleanse; its humectant attribute helps to hold natural moisture on skin without the introduction of oil.

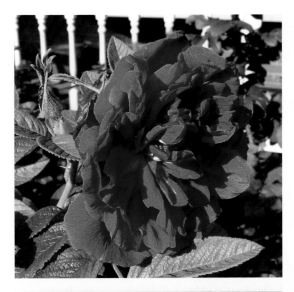

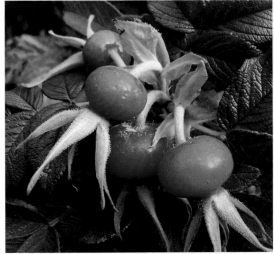

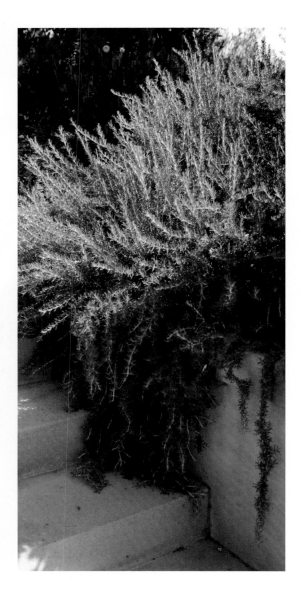

■ Rosemary

Common Name: Rosemary

Botanical Name: *Rosemarinus officinalis*

Culture: USDA Zone 7. Tender perennial treated as an annual below Zone 7. The trailing rosemary *R. officinalis* 'Prostratus Group' is not hardy at all below Zone 7. The upright variety *R. officinalis* 'Arp' has been proven to be the hardiest and is known to overwinter in Zone 5. Needs full sun and well-draining soil. Place in a warm spot near rockery and walls that gather heat from the sun.

Properties: Aromatic, antifungal, stimulating

Parts used: Leaves, fresh and dried.

Notes: Strong pine-like fragrance, a favorite in culinary dishes. The leaves steeped in water are used as a skin cleanser and deep hair rinse for brunettes. Rosemary is a "wake-up" herb because of its heavy, enchanting fragrance; the volatile essential oil on the fresh leaves in the peak of summer will linger on your hands after rubbing it. Use in bath blends, hair mixes and cleansing balms.

Sage

Common Name: Sage, garden sage

Botanical Name: *Salvia officinalis*

Culture: Zone hardiness varies by variety and is typically hardy to USDA Zone 4. Shrubby and herbaceous perennials. Growth varies from 6 inches to 3 feet, based on variety. Common garden sage *(Salvia officinalis)* is the best for cosmetic use; the leaf color and texture of golden sage *(S. officinalis* 'Aurea'), purple sage *(S. officinalis* 'Purpurea') and Berggarten sage *(S. officinalis* 'Berggarten') make them an attractive addition to an herb garden.

Properties: Astringent, stimulating, cleansing.

Parts Used: Leaves, fresh and dried.

Notes: Rich, earthy fragrance. Highly astringent for cleaning up oily, dirty skin. Strong disinfectant, good to mix in spray mists with lavender and mints. A hair rinse made with sage will darken hair color and make hair smooth and shiny. In topical skin care it is very useful for oily and irritated skin.

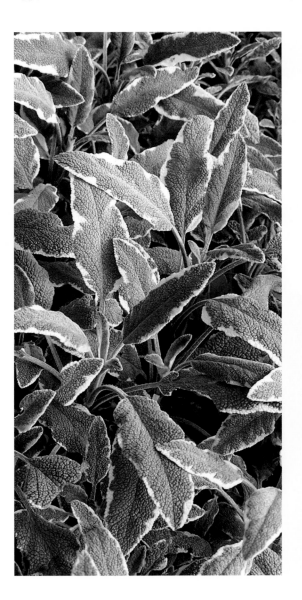

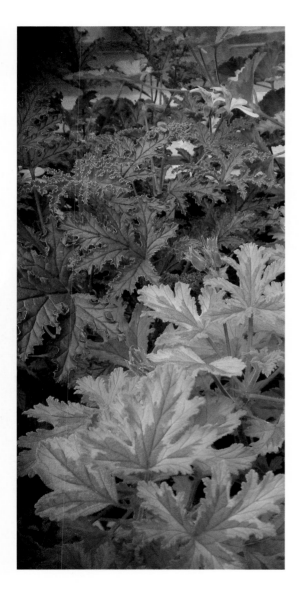

▪ Scented Geranium

Common Name: Scented geranium, scented leaf geranium

Botanical Name: *Pelargonium*

Culture: USDA Zone 10. Tender shrubby plant. Protect from frost. Needs full sun and well-draining soil. Grows up to 3 feet in height. In colder climates, grow as an annual or in containers that can be protected in the winter.

Properties: Mild astringent, anti-aging, anti-fungal

Parts Used: Leaves, use fresh and dried

Notes: In historical herbals it is said that geraniums planted around the home will keep evil spirits away. The rich, aromatic leaves of scented geraniums release fragrance when brushed against. Most of the species in the genus of scented-leaf pelargoniums have astringent properties. The rose scented varieties are the most widely used for medicinal and culinary purposes: rose geranium *(Pelargonium graveolens)*, 'Attar of Roses' *(P. capitatum)*, 'Lady Plymouth' *(P. graveolens variegata)*. The oil from *Pelargonium graveolens* is reputed to have skin healing properties and popular for use in aromatherapy practice as an anti-depressant.

▪ Thyme

Common Name: Thyme

Botanical Name: *Thymus* spp.

Culture: USDA Zone 4. Full sun, low growing (under 12 inches) herbaceous perennial. Will stay evergreen in mild winter areas. Tolerates dry, rocky soils.

Properties: Antiseptic, stimulating

Parts Used: Leaves, fresh and dried

Notes: The upright thymes, such as English and French thyme *(Thymus vulgaris)*, lemon thyme *(T. x citriodorus)* and silver thyme *(T. vulgaris* 'Argenteus'), are all highly fragrant varieties that grow full for good leaf production. In history, thyme was popular in purification rituals and embalming, attributed to the antiseptic qualities of the essential oil present in the leaves and stems.

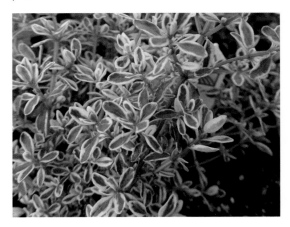

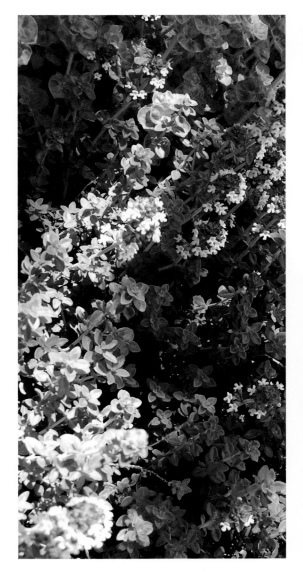

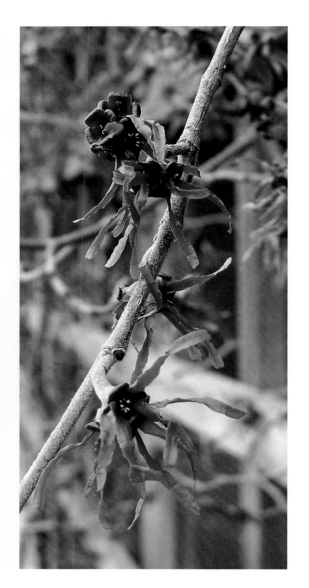

▪ Witch Hazel

Common Name: Witch Hazel

Botanical Name: *Hamamelis* spp.

Culture: USDA Zone 3. Deciduous shrub. Grows up to 10 feet. Prefers moist, well-drained soil in part shade. The blooms cover the branches in late winter before the leaves appear.

Properties: Astringent, soothing

Parts Used: Bark, leaves

Notes: *Hamamelis virginiana* is native to the eastern United States and Canada. Long revered as a healing plant by Native Americans, the leaves were used as a topical poultice to ease swelling. An extract distilled in alcohol from fresh leaves and young twigs is commonly used as a skin tonic to soothe and heal. For spa and skin care, use true witch hazel extract, found in natural food markets, which will have a lower percentage of alcohol than the commercial witch hazel you find in the drug store. (See page 126 for more about witch hazel.)

DESIGNING AND GROWING:
4 SEASONS IN THE GARDEN AND CONTAINERS

Whether your herb garden is large and ornate or small and contained, there's a place to grow fresh herbs. They will give back in so many ways.

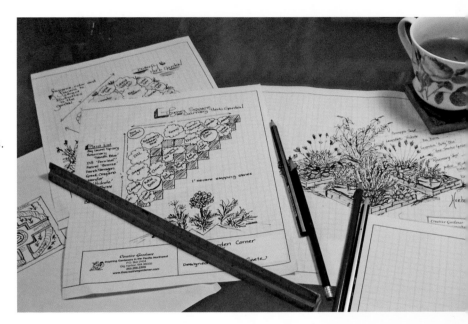

In the planning of an herb garden, it is important to remember just what the garden is for: it is for an abundant harvest. This means good growing conditions but also easy ways to access the plants for harvest. Place the garden where it is easy to get to. Remember, you will be cutting handfuls or even large bundles and taking them in to use. Don't place the herb plot so far out or hard to access that you are exhausted just getting out to it.

Consider Design

Grow creatively to add interest in all seasons. Herb gardens are spaces that will always be cut and harvested from. Defining a permanent framework for herbs will allow plants to come and go without taking away from the design and

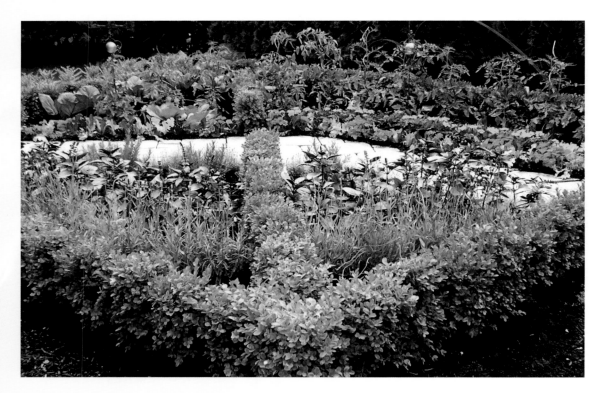

having the herbs' off-season be ugly. Start your design by drawing lines – enclose, circle or create squares and rectangles to form space for your plantings. Play with patterning. Maximize the design of an herb garden by planting artistically. That could mean re-thinking straight rows – laying out garden beds with creative patterns that intermingle with each other, reminiscent of small knot gardens. Fringe walkways with parsley. Serpentine a row of variegated lemon thyme through a flowerbed or create geometric shapes of bush basil around upright rosemary. *Tip:* Be sure your pathways give easy access (at least 3 feet wide.)

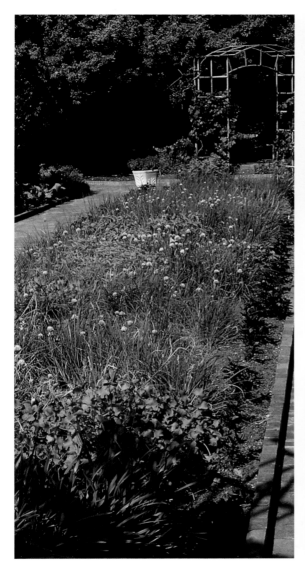

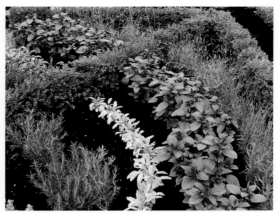

"With few exceptions the herbs are not endowed with conspicuous or brilliantly colored flowers. Theirs is a modest beauty, appreciated by gardeners long at their work who have learned to enjoy the less obvious and more subtle qualities in plants…"

Helen M. Fox, *Gardening with Herbs*, 1933.

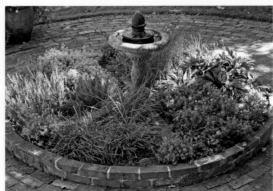

Planting

Start the garden with healthy soil; introduce compost or other amendments into garden beds to create a well-draining, rich environment. Most of the plants in this book do well in well-draining, humus-rich soil, full of natural nutrients. Loosen soil to a depth of 10 to 12 inches before planting.

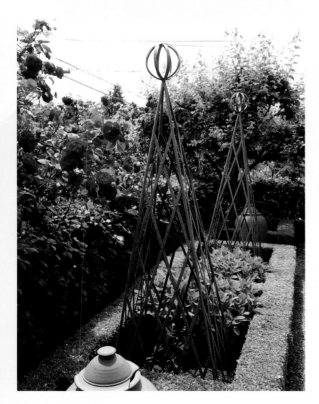

Herbs do best in full sun or a good quality of sun for most of the day. Many herbs are native to Mediterranean regions of the world and thrive in heat and light. Look for micro-climates in the garden where heat and light gather, such as near brick or stone walls.

Plant annuals by seed or transplants when soil is warmed and after the last frost in your area, typically in the month of May. Hardy perennials can be planted as soon as the soil is workable (not sloppy or muddy) in the spring.

5 Herbal Habits to Know:

- Some do well from seed: basil, borage, calendula, chamomile, parsley
- Some are better from cuttings: hops, lavender, lemon balm, lemon verbena, mint, pelargoniums, rosemary, sage, thyme
- Some are best as a rooted, healthy plant: eucalyptus, rose, witch hazel
- Some are rampant spreaders (be wary!): borage, hops, lemon balm, mint
- And some you just can't seem to have enough of (plant plentifully!): basil, lemon verbena

Herbal Knot Trio

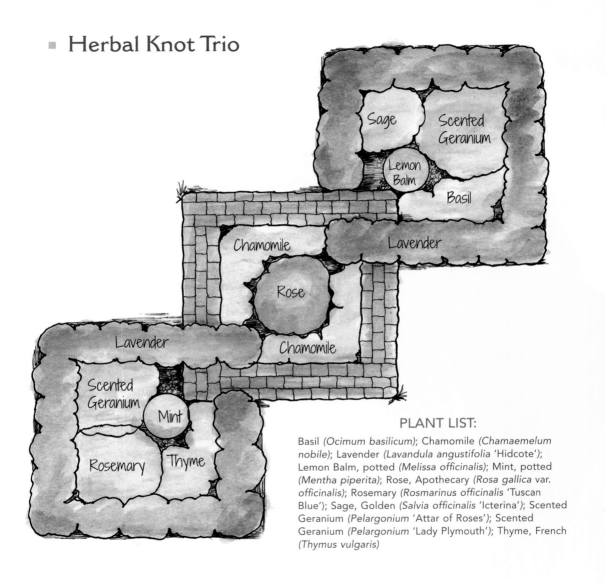

Sage

Scented
Geranium

Lemon
Balm

Basil

Chamomile

Lavender

Rose

Chamomile

Lavender

Scented
Geranium

Mint

Rosemary

Thyme

PLANT LIST:

Basil *(Ocimum basilicum)*; Chamomile *(Chamaemelum nobile)*; Lavender *(Lavandula angustifolia* 'Hidcote'*)*; Lemon Balm, potted *(Melissa officinalis)*; Mint, potted *(Mentha piperita)*; Rose, Apothecary *(Rosa gallica* var. *officinalis)*; Rosemary *(Rosmarinus officinalis* 'Tuscan Blue'*)*; Sage, Golden *(Salvia officinalis* 'Icterina'*)*; Scented Geranium *(Pelargonium* 'Attar of Roses'*)*; Scented Geranium *(Pelargonium* 'Lady Plymouth'*)*; Thyme, French *(Thymus vulgaris)*

■ Herbal Squares ■

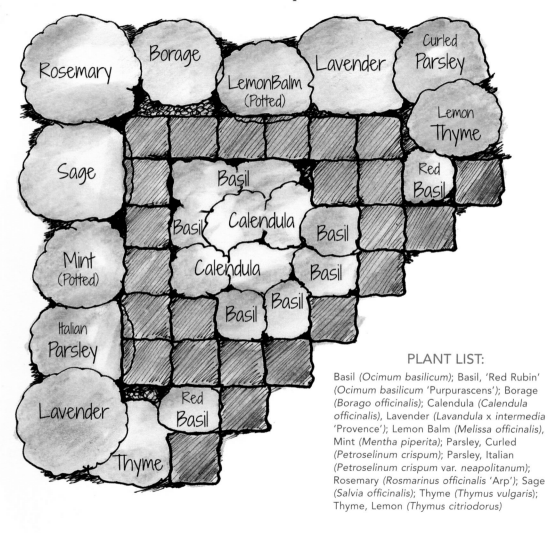

Rosemary

Borage

LemonBalm
(Potted)

Lavender

Curled
Parsley

Lemon
Thyme

Sage

Basil

Basil

Calendula

Red
Basil

Basil

Mint
(Potted)

Calendula

Basil

Basil

Italian
Parsley

Basil

Basil

Lavender

Red
Basil

Thyme

PLANT LIST:

Basil *(Ocimum basilicum)*; Basil, 'Red Rubin' *(Ocimum basilicum 'Purpurascens')*; Borage *(Borago officinalis)*; Calendula *(Calendula officinalis)*, Lavender *(Lavandula × intermedia 'Provence')*; Lemon Balm *(Melissa officinalis)*, Mint *(Mentha piperita)*; Parsley, Curled *(Petroselinum crispum)*; Parsley, Italian *(Petroselinum crispum var. neapolitanum)*; Rosemary *(Rosmarinus officinalis 'Arp')*; Sage *(Salvia officinalis)*; Thyme *(Thymus vulgaris)*; Thyme, Lemon *(Thymus citriodorus)*

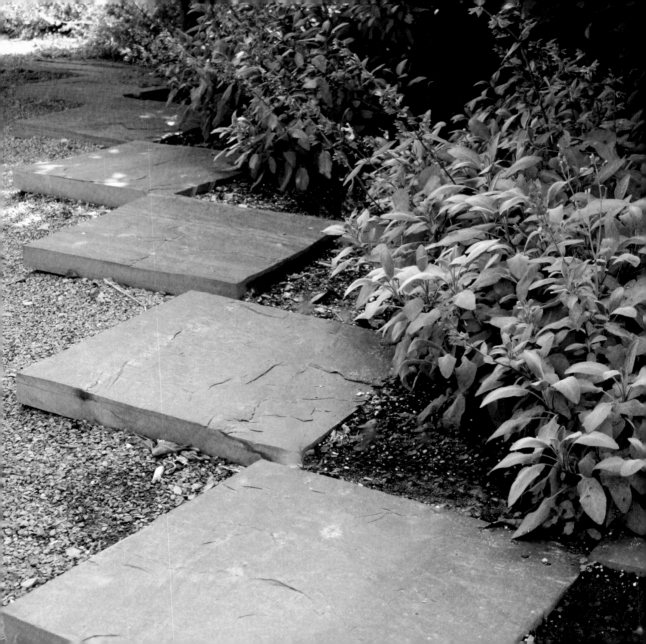

Herbal Spa Garden

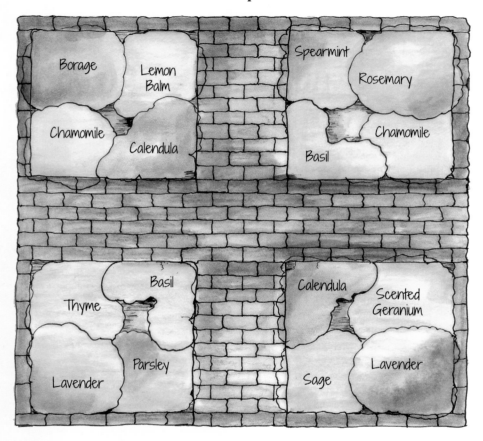

PLANT LIST:

Basil *(Ocimum basilicum 'Genovese')*; Borage *(Borago officinalis)*; Chamomile *(Matricaria recutita 'Bodegold')*; Calendula *(Calendula officinalis)*; Lavender *(Lavandula angustifolia 'Provence')*; Lemon Balm *(Melissa officinalis)*; Scented Geranium, rose *(Pelargonium graveolens)*; Spearmint *(Mentha spicata)*; Parsley *(Petroselinum crispum)*; Rosemary *(Rosmarinus officinalis 'Blue Spires')*; Sage *(Salvia officinalis)*; Thyme, silver *(Thymus vulgaris 'Argenteus')*

HERBS CONTAINED!

Growing outdoors in containers is a stylish, easy way to add herbs to a garden space. Pottery introduces the decorative touch while the herbs offer their unique fragrance, flavor and texture to the plantings. For some gardeners, container plantings are the only option to grow a garden and for others they become points of creative artistry in large spaces. Containers have no limits beyond their actual size and shape. They can be placed almost anywhere and become an instant garden where none existed before.

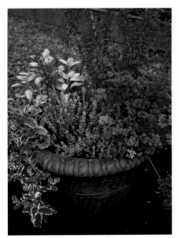

Herbs in containers also give versatility for fragrant and edible gardening on a balcony, patio, or a space where it is not easy to grow in the ground. Plants in pots are portable. The simple fact is that small gardens are small maintenance; no weeding, mowing, raking, edging. The low maintenance aspect of container growing makes this is one of the easiest types of garden to grow.

Containers with style

Choosing the right container is as important as choosing the right plants to grow in them. Glazed, embossed, elegant, textural, heavy, light, contemporary, or traditional; the choice of pot can be the style maker. Creating atmosphere, adding artistry and style can all be done with container gardens. Think of the container as an important part of the whole look you are trying to create. If the theme or mood calls for a real terra cotta pot then use one; an imitation plastic one will never look right. If the color of the home, patio furniture or other things will be in direct view of the pot, then coordinate the effort. Remember, the colors of pottery are not seasonal; a color clash will never go away.

The plants

The mixture of plants or individually potted plants grouped together can make or break a good container garden setting. Don't be afraid to try out different combinations. Plants that have the same cultural needs, such as shade, sun or heavy moisture, should be planted together. Plants that are aggressive and fast growing, like mints and lemon balm should be planted by themselves.

Care and keeping of herbs in containers

Use the right size for what is being grown in the pot. Balance the mature height and width of plants to the dimensions of the pot. Water drainage through containers is an absolute must. Make sure the container has a drainage hole and the soil is not compacted. An inch or two of loose gravel or broken pieces of terra cotta at the bottom of the container will help keep the drainage hole open so water can flow out.

Water containers when dry, and avoid over-watering, especially drought tolerant herbs like rosemary or lavender. How much water depends on the weather, the plant's requirements and the type of pot. Pots can dry quickly in the heat of the summer, so check often and water as needed.

Potting soil: go for good old-fashioned organic mixes. Good soil makes good drainage. You can top dress with finished compost over the seasons to add back natural nutrients.

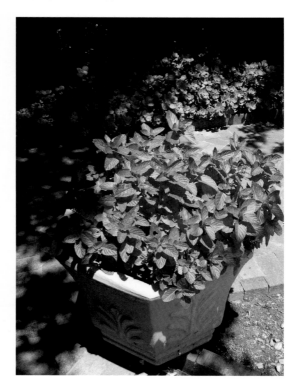

GROW A WINDOWSILL GARDEN

Brighten up a sunny window with potted herbs and use fresh herbs through the winter. Some good varieties for potted indoor gardens: basil, lemon balm, mint, parsley, rosemary, sage, scented geraniums and thyme. Place potted herbs in a sunny window. Herbs prefer temperatures around 70 degrees F. Make sure the windowsill doesn't get lower than 45 degrees F. at night in the cooler months of the year. Plant in well-draining pottery. Terra cotta pots work well because they are porous and help keep roots from remaining too wet. Just remember that terra cotta also tends to dry out faster. Lightly mist them daily to provide humidity; don't saturate the leaves with droplets. Check the soil moisture and water only when they are just starting to dry out, and be careful not to over-water. When watering in the winter, treat herbs to tepid water, instead of a cold shower.

Harvest regularly to keep herbs from overtaking their space in the window.

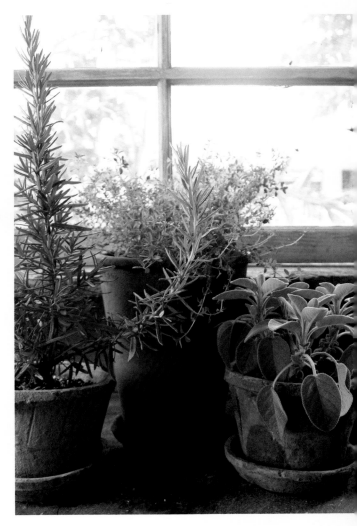

SEASONAL TASKS IN THE HERB GARDEN

Herbs in the garden are some of the easiest plants to care for. They don't require a lot but do need seasonal care. In any garden there are tasks to be done. One of the best tools for an easy care garden is to simply do seasonal tasks as needed rather than have the work of a garden overwhelm. The small tasks left undone over a few season become larger and problematic. Keeping an eye out for disease and pests, pruning them in the correct season, clean-up and taking care of the cultural needs, such as good soil – all are good habits of a sustainable garden.

Keeping an Herb Garden Calendar

A garden diary or calendar helps to keep track of plants, tasks and yearly occurrences. Write down actual planting dates, bloom time, pruning and harvest dates of herbs. Some oddities of plant growth can be attributed to when a late freeze hit – or a sudden heat wave at a period of growth in the plant. It is as simple as getting an ordinary calendar that has blocks for each day where you can leave a note. Journal something every day about the garden – air temperature, rain, frost, a garden task completed for the day. It may even be a bird sighting or a new bloom that opened up. Whether it is ritual or out of the ordinary, make note of it on the day it

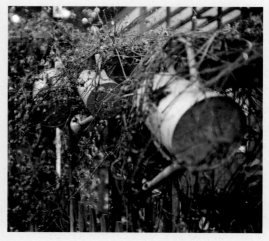

occurred. This is a great tool to give you an overview of your gardening year – and to make plans for the upcoming year.

Spring

■ Spring is the time to give gardens a good cleanup. Remove winter debris and, as weather permits, the winter mulch from on top of plants. Prune broken branches, clip off old seed heads and stem remnants from perennials.

■ Keep an eye out for pests and disease. The best plan is to notice problems before they cause major damage (of course!). Ongoing observation is a good tool. As weather warms, aphids, scale and spider mites get active. Control slugs and snails.

■ Top dress planting beds and perennial container gardens with compost. In arid climates and high desert zones, mulch will help retain moisture on the surface. Replace soil in empty container gardens to insure there are no overwintering disease or pests.

■ Amend soil. Organic compost adds nutrients and humus.

■ Plant hardy perennial herbs like sage and thyme when the ground is not frozen or muddy.

■ Shear lavender and other woody herbs when small leaf buds appear in the woody part of the plants. Based on the size and shape, they can be trimmed by a third if needed.

■ Look at plants that have overgrown their space or are stealing beauty from other plants. Remove or properly prune as needed.

■ Rake and lightly mow low-growing groundcover herbs like chamomile.

Summer

■ Keep ahead of weeds. Have small weed-pulling sessions before plants flower and drop seed, instead of letting them overwhelm you with work.

■ Clip faded blossoms of annuals, perennials, and shrub roses to encourage new bud formation.

■ Stay on pest patrol. Fungus (like powdery mildew) and insects like warm weather; populations can break out almost overnight.

■ Freshen container gardens with a layer of new soil on top. Add summer color with herbs like calendula. Add foliage texture with purple garden sage, curly parsley, and burgundy leaf basils.

■ When nighttime temperatures are reliably above 50 degrees F., basil can go out in the garden and in containers.

Fall

■ Continue keeping plants tidy as they finish their summer abundance. Plants that have over-bloomed and are falling over need to be removed so they don't harm other plants.

■ Fall compost can be added as needed to top dress beds for the end of the season.

■ Lift and divide spring blooming perennial herbs.

■ Trim faded blooms off of lavender, but do not cut into the woody parts of the plants. Tidy the plants into a neat mushroom-shaped mound.

■ Know your first average frost date and keep an eye on the weather report; if frost threatens, harvest herbs for drying before they are damaged.

■ Protect tender plants for winter. Mulch at the correct time for your area. Too early and it will artificially keep the soil warm and keep plants from a natural dormancy. Too late and the plants may have already been damaged. A good rule of thumb is to apply mulch when weather reaches a freezing point and stays cold. In mild climates, zone 6 and above, most herbs don't need a winter blanket of mulch for warmth.

■ Photograph any mixed borders or areas that may need plant additions. Use them for reference for winter and early spring garden planning.

Winter

■ In hard winter areas after the ground freezes and snow begins, enjoy the slower pace of the garden and dream of designs for next year. Collect ideas and plants to look for to add to the garden. Learn about new herbs to introduce.

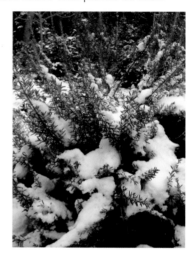

■ Pile snow, pine needles, evergreen boughs or straw on the crowns of susceptible perennials for winter protection from freezing, desiccating winds.

■ In mild climate zones stay on weed watch for perennial weeds and early annuals like chickweed.

■ Prune deciduous trees and shrubs if needed while dormant, when you can see their branching habits.

■ On nice weather days, clean up storm damage debris and trim broken branches to prevent further damage.

HARVESTING AND PRESERVING
(DRYING, FREEZING)

Harvesting

Herbs are at the most flavorful and fragrant in the morning after the dew dries. This is the best time to pick. If the herbs are dirty, you may want to water them lightly to clean them the day before you pick. It helps the herbs not to lose their precious oils and not get soggy if you don't have to wash them after picking.

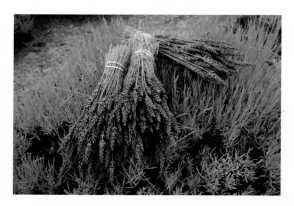

Quick Tips for Fresh Harvesting in Growing Season

Do not cut more than one-third off of perennials. Leave at least 6 inches or a minimum of half the plant on annuals. The plants need to have enough leaves and fresh growth left behind to continue to grow through the remaining season.

Don't pluck or pull them; use scissors to cut the plants cleanly without damaging them.

Leaves: Young leaves have the highest amount of flavor and fragrance, so harvest these as needed. Most plants have a flush of green just before they flower. Cut and harvest them so the oils will not be lost to the flowers.

Flowers: Harvest just as the plant begins to flower and harvest no later than its peak of flowering or the look and taste will fade.

Seeds: Pick just before they fully ripen, cut the stalks and tie into bundles. Invert inside a brown paper bag and hang. As the seeds dry they will fall into the bag to can be shaken to loosen them in the bag.

YOUR STILLROOM

Gardens in the early American colonies were not for ornamentation; they were planted and worked with for food in season and preserving for the off-season. Specific plants were grown to provide food, soaps, perfumes, insecticides, dyes, and medicines – all the things needed to take care of everyday life in the home. The luxury of going to the corner drugstore to buy necessities did not exist. Remedies were mixed and blended on site. Every good sustainable homestead had an herb garden that supplied its own pharmacopoeia. In the home, a "stillroom," typically off the kitchen, was set aside to prepare household products from the garden. This was where cosmetics, medicine, bathing and laundry products were created and distilled. The space emitted earthy aromas of fresh-cut flowers and drying herb bundles hung from the ceiling.

As the industrial revolution progressed, many households became able to purchase items commercially, leaving less need for a stillroom. In our lifestyle today, the fragrant storage room of preserved plants is not typical, but the methods of a stillroom are being revived. The lost art of the stillroom is coming back, thanks to our fascination with gardens and how they give back to us with food, healing remedies and body care products. I hope you can find a space to store your harvests so that at any time of the year you can have the ingredients ready for you – mint for a reviving foot soak, lavender to soothe your skin, lemon verbena for a steamy facial, chamomile flowers for your herbal sleep pillow.

PRESERVING

Gathering herbs at the end of the season is vital to keeping supplies available after the garden has gone quiet for the winter. To get the best of the garden in the preservation process, take good care to harvest at the right time and dry the plant materials carefully.

■ As with fresh harvesting through the growing season, it is best to harvest them in the morning after the dew dries.

■ When the summer wanes and fall begins, keep an eye on herbaceous perennials that are fading. Harvest herbs when they still look good and not when the foliage is drying or turning brown.

■ Keep watch on the weather and as first frost is approaching, make sure to harvest any tender or annual plants before they are killed by the cold.

The time you take at harvest and preserving is part of your own quality control and will provide you with herbs in every month of the year.

■ Consider the shelf life of dried or frozen herbs as "harvest to harvest."

Use up herbs before the next season is harvested so the supply is never more than a year old.

■ Store dried herb in glass jars and keep in a cabinet away from sun and heat.

■ Label all the jars with the herb name and harvest date, herbs look alike after they are dried.

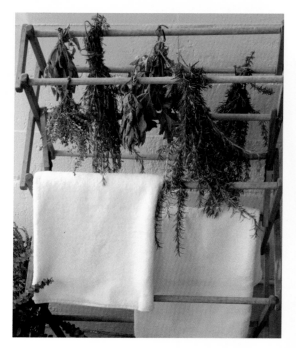

Hang dry

This is the most popular way to preserve herbs from the garden.

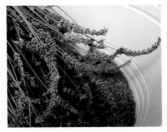

What to do: Dry them in a dark, airy place. Make sure they are not in direct sunlight and have good air circulation around them. Bundle them with rubber bands and hang them upside down. To remove leaves or flowers from dried stems, simply strip the dried plants from the stems or shake into a paper bag until the stems are cleaned, then empty the bag into a spice jar. Leaves and seeds should be kept whole, to be crushed down when needed.

Freeze

An alternative to drying herbs is to freeze them. Some, not all, herbs will retain their properties when frozen. The freezing process will darken leaves and change the look of the herbs, but will hardly be noticeable when blended into mixes or added into hot liquids.

Herbs that will freeze well:

Basil
Parsley
Lemon verbena
Mint

What to do: Harvest and rinse in cool water and pat dry. Remove the leaves and flowers from the stiff stems. Use sharp scissors and cut them up. Sprinkle them over a cookie sheet and put them in the freezer for about an hour. Put in freezer bags and return to the freezer. This method allows you to sprinkle them into recipes instead of freezing them in a big clump.

Easy herbal ice cubes:

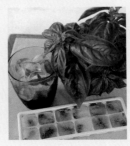

Put 1 teaspoon or 1 fresh leaf of an herb into each square of an ice cube tray and fill with water. When frozen, pop the cubes out and store them in freezer bags. The ice cubes can be melted to use in recipes calling for a specific herb water.

PART THREE

CREATE

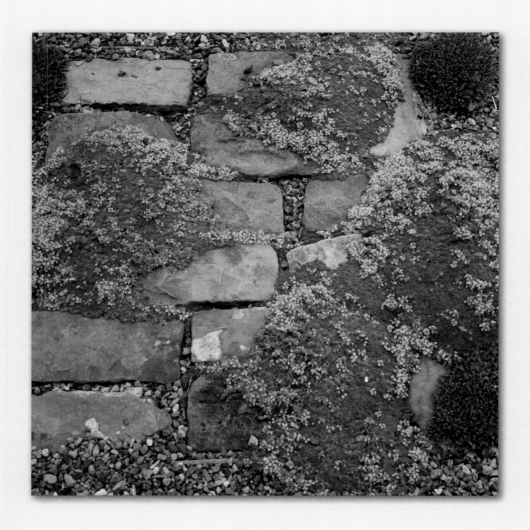

When we dig deeper into the nature of the garden,

we come to the realm of

healing and nurturing the body.

Plants are our oldest form of medicine; many medicines we use today are based on recipes used thousands of years ago. In the study of cultures we find many stories that speak of human interaction with plants…legends and lore about spiritual healing as well as physical healing. It is fascinating to learn how certain plants were discovered and became valued for these qualities. Nature herself begs us to discover her gifts by luring us with fragrance, flavor, color and feel. When we garden, we connect with all of those senses. Perhaps the most familiar use of plants is for flavor, the sense of taste. Growing food is a common thread that connects us back to the earth. Gardeners relish the first taste of a fresh tomato off

the vine or a strawberry oozing with juice. And we love our herbs for adding zest to our food; in the garden it is their fragrance that first enchants us. We can experience an aromatherapy treatment simply by brushing past a rosemary bush or walking barefoot on a thyme-filled path.

What is it about herbs that affects us so positively when we incorporate them into our spa rituals? On one level, the subtle essences of the plants grasp and manipulate our brain functions, producing feelings of relaxation, of stimulation, of overall wellbeing. On another level, we experience the healing properties of the herbs themselves when they are applied directly to the skin.

In this part of our book I offer some of my favorite recipes, with notes, tips and ideas to aid you in embracing the use of herbs in your home spa. Think of it as your personal spa compendium.

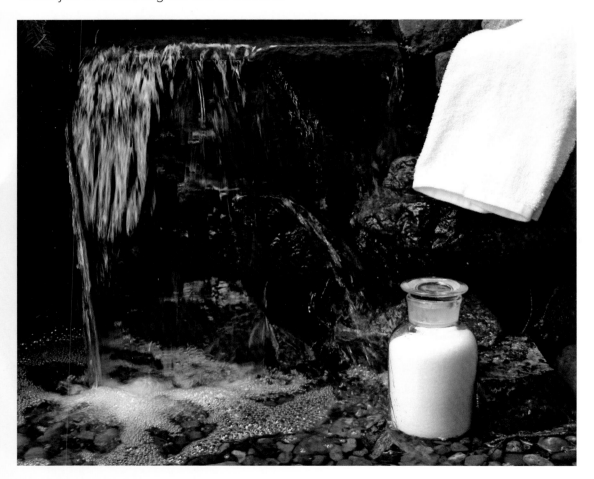

HOMEMADE NOTES

(all about your ingredients and how to prepare them)

Fresh-from-the-garden spa treatments will be very different from the products you see on the shelves at the corner drug store. Home blended recipes do not rely on ingredients (those long letter, unpronounceable words you see listed on the bottle of commercially produced items) that preserve, color or help stabilize the consistency. So when your homemade products look and behave differently from the heavily enhanced commercial products, rejoice – you're getting your treatments direct from the source, the way nature intended.

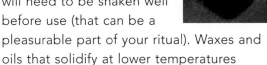

The natural, raw state of herbs infused into liquids or waxes may be grainy with plant sediment. Oils and waters will separate and will need to be shaken well before use (that can be a pleasurable part of your ritual). Waxes and oils that solidify at lower temperatures should be warmed before use. Colors will often be an earthy shade of beige or brown; the use of some plants, like the golden color of pot marigold (*Calendula officinalis*), will bring their natural colors to the ingredients they are infused into.

It is important to remember that your recipes will not have preservatives. Herbs added to water begin to quickly break down, making the mix rancid within a matter of days, because bacteria and fungus love to grow in water. Oils will also become rancid over time due to oxidation. However, natural ingredients with high levels of sugar, salt, alcohol or vinegar will have some preservative qualities when added to water and oil mixes. So you can see that the shelf life of your recipes and ingredients can vary tremendously, depending on a number of factors – including heat, sunlight and air. Add to this the chemistry of nature and microbes, and the science experiment begins!

Be Kind to Yourself and Mother Earth
(sourcing your ingredients)

Just as you do with the food you eat, consider the source of the herbs and ingredients you use for your spa creations. Purchase from merchants who buy from farmers who use sustainable growing practices. Source from suppliers who follow the concerns of the marketplace and practice environmental stewardship in how they choose their line of products.

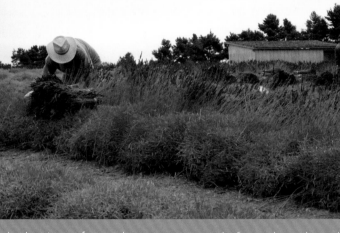

For spices, oils and other items from other countries, look for Fair Trade. This is not just a label, it is a practice that means farmers and producers are treated and paid fairly.

Some herbs and natural products are harvested from the wild. Try to make sure that a product was ethically harvested or wild crafted with responsibility to the land.

By making homemade preparations you are the quality control expert. You make the choice for freshness and purity, and sourcing ingredients is an important part of the process. And by cutting out the commercial manufacturing and packaging you are helping the environment by not adding to the waste stream. When sourcing your ingredients, choose base oils made from fruits and nuts instead of petroleum-based oils such as mineral or baby oil.

Always grow and source plants by organic means. Buy organic seeds and plants and grow them chemical free. Remember that what goes in the garden soil and on plants goes into your body when you apply it to your skin.

COMMON INGREDIENTS TO KNOW

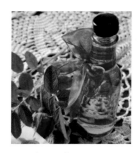

Alcohol: (natural grain alcohols): used as a preservative or carrier for herbs.

Apple cider vinegar: astringent, restores pH on skin. Use natural apple cider vinegar or "living vinegar" purchased at natural health food markets.

Do not use white vinegar in body care treatments; it is too harsh on skin.

Avocado: used for its meat, made into pulp. Conditioning to hair and skin, high in vitamins A and E.

Beeswax: a natural wax, an emulsifier. Slight sweet fragrance adds a tinge of yellow to balms and salves. Purchase from a local beekeeper.

How to Measure Beeswax

Most beeswax is available in solid blocks. When a recipe calls for an amount, it can be challenging to know if the amount you can shave off a brick will be enough for the recipe. To use, grate or slice off the block in small pieces – or make up a batch of premeasured pieces in a double boiler or the microwave.

Double boiler method: Slowly melt the wax until it is liquid. Pour into a tablespoon measuring spoon and allow to harden (putting it in the freezer for a minute will speed up the process). Store the premeasured wax pieces in a jar or bag.

Microwave method: In a glass microwave-safe bowl, add cut or grated pieces of beeswax. Place in the

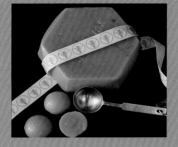

microwave for 30 seconds and check it. Stir with a bamboo skewer to help the larger pieces melt. Be patient! Continue to warm at 30-second intervals until the wax is liquid. Pour into spoons as noted above.

Baking soda (sodium bicarbonate): balances skin pH, acid neutralizer. Good for itchy, irritated skin and also helps draw out impurities.

Castile soap: made from vegetable fat, not animal fat. It is a gentle basic soap, typically available in liquid form that can be infused with herbs to create personal, signature blends of shower soap or shampoo.

Cheesecloth: a natural loose weave cloth that is used to filter herbs and other sediment from liquids. Use 100% organic cotton.

Cocoa butter: a hard wax-like substance at room temperature, but easily melts on skin. Slight chocolate fragrance. This is a fatty wax that softens skin.

Coconut oil: a mild, non-fragrant oil that remains solid until it reaches about 75 degrees F. Quickly melts on skin. Good addition to scrubs and massage oils. Suspends bulky herbs for use in a solid, spreadable form.

Cornmeal: ground corn that adds texture to scrubs to exfoliate dead cells from the surface of skin.

Cornstarch: finely ground corn. An absorbent powder material used to help soothe and dry skin.

Cucumber: the quintessential image of a spa facial: sliced cucumbers placed over the eyes. This vegetable is a cleansing agent that reduces puffiness and is soothing and healing to delicate skin, particularly the delicate folds of skin around eyes.

Epsom salt (magnesium sulfate): draws toxins out of the skin, soothes muscle and joint aches. Water softener that neutralizes pH. (For more about salt, see page 120.)

Essential oils: an extraction of oils from plant tissues. (See page 108.)

Grape seed oil: light green base-carrier oil. Good oil for massage and bathing. Light, non-greasy, fragrance-free with a very low allergen quality.

Ginger root: the rhizome of *Zingiber officinale*. Purchase roots and use fresh grated in body care recipes. Ginger is a warming spice that detoxes the body by promoting sweating.

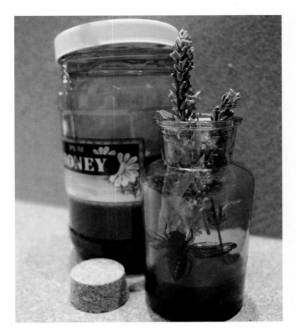

Honey: used as a skin softener and also as a sweetener for drinking tea.

To make herb-infused honey: Fill a clean glass pint-size canning jar ½ full with fresh or dried herbs. Pour honey (use local, fresh raw honey) to the top of the jar, leaving about an inch of head space. Cover. Place honey/herb jar in a pan of water on the stove and allow the honey to warm (do not boil). The warmth will help release the essential oils of the herbs. Remove from heat and allow to sit for a week. Strain out the herb and place in a clean jar. Cover tightly. Honey also acts as a natural preservative due to its high sugar content.

Jojoba oil: a base-carrier oil. Good conditioner for skin, scalp and hair. It has an excellent reputation as a base oil because it is technically a liquid ester, which is an oily substance very close to the makeup of natural skin oils. Good all-purpose carrier with a long shelf life.

Lemon and lime: fragrant and acidic fruits. The juice restores pH and is mildly bleaching to skin. The zest from the skin adds astringent qualities, coloring and texture.

Muslin: 100% cotton fabric with a tighter weave. Use unbleached muslin for bath bags and sachets. Also can be used as a filter to strain herbs out of liquids.

Oats, oatmeal (whole, natural): skin exfoliant. Adds natural skin softening to water and liquid blends. (For more on oats, see page 111.)

Rice flour: uncooked rice, ground into a fine powder. Used for body powders and as a base to make paste for face masks.

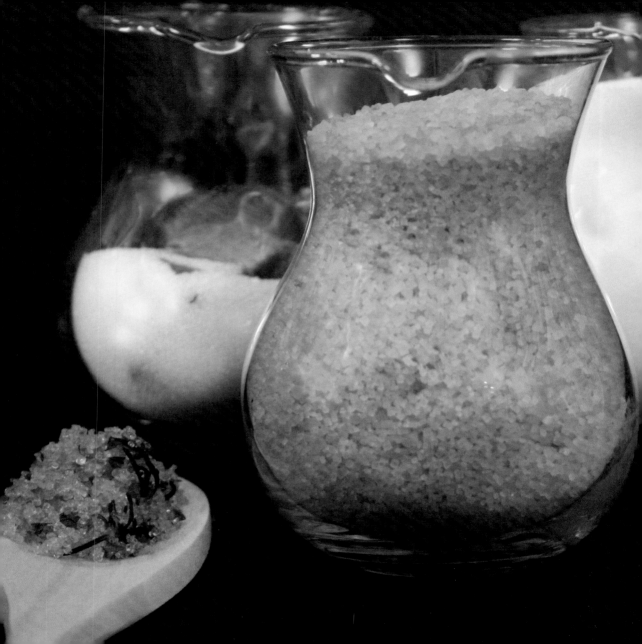

Sea salt: natural water softener. Popular as an exfoliant. Use fine-ground in bath salts to easily dissolve. Larger, coarser grinds are useful for scrubs on tougher skin like hands and feet. (For more about types of salt, see page 120.)

Sugars: good exfoliant in scrubs. Use natural organic raw, washed or coconut sugar.

Sweet almond oil: a good basic base carrier oil, for all skin types. High in fatty acids makes it good for restoring softness to skin. Has a limited shelf life; use opened bottles within 6 months.

Vanilla bean: the fruit of an orchid grown in temperate climates. It is one of the more expensive spices and is used to flavor lip balms and scent lotions and oils. Seeds scraped from the inside of the pods are used in scrubs, bath salts, oils and soap.

Vitamin E oil: acts as a natural preservative to slow oxidation of lotions, oils and balms. Healing and moisturizing. Use only 100% natural d-alpha tocopherol to avoid synthetic versions of this common vitamin.

Vodka: plant-derived alcohol base to preserve herbs. Use as a tincture base and in toner recipes. Use 100 proof, if available, because it has little to no fragrance to interact with the herbs aromas. Also good for cleansing storage equipment by removing oily residue from metal and glass.

Water: distilled or pure spring water, not tap water.

Witch hazel: cleanses pores and tightens skin. (See page 126.)

Yogurt (plain): skin softener, mildly astringent.

Herb Measurement Guidelines

All are approximate, based on common varieties and harvest methods.

1 ounce equals:

1/2 cup powdered (like cornstarch)

3/4 cup fine or small dried (like lavender buds)

1 cup bulky dried (calendula flowers, lemon verbena leaves)

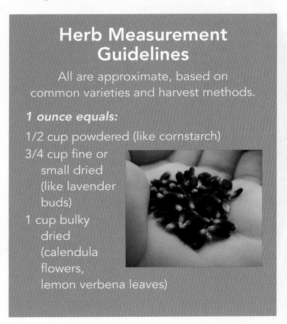

DECONSTRUCTING AN HERBAL RECIPE

(the importance of knowing your ingredients and what they do)

I know there is a lot of information available to you about making fresh herbal goodies from the garden. Some of that information is excellent and some has not proven its worth – so how do we know if an herbal recipe is a good one? It all comes down to the ingredient mix.

I tend to think through (maybe even over-think) the individual ingredients that make up a recipe. I am interested in knowing why there is salt in a chocolate chip cookie recipe or baking soda in biscuits. The point is, knowing what each ingredient does to make the whole. Body care recipes are the same as culinary ones. If you get to know each ingredient, you know the way it works and the benefits of having it in the recipe.

We can find a lot of information just by typing on the computer: ideas, tips and do-it-yourself projects, in numerous forms and from many sources. Make information an asset

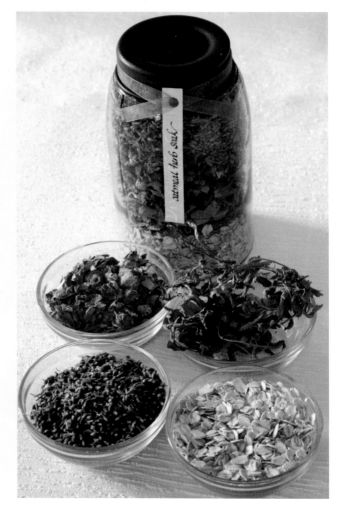

by finding resources that will help you learn what you need to know about herbs and their properties. And become savvy about the other ingredients that help you get the herbs into a usable form. When you recognize the individual ingredients, you understand the healing and nurturing qualities of an herbal body care recipe.

For example, let's deconstruct the Calendula Salve recipe in the Winter Solstice section (page 158). It calls for using calendula petals, avocado or olive oil, beeswax and Vitamin E oil. The herb calendula is used for its reputation for healing and soothing irritated skin. The avocado oil "carries" or has been infused with the qualities of the calendula. The beeswax gives the infused herbal oil a texture that helps it penetrate into skin; the wax also gives a natural protection barrier from outside elements. The Vitamin E oil preserves the calendula (which can be affected by heat and light). Vitamin E also adds its own level of skin restorative qualities. Pretty simple!

The takeaway I want you to remember is this: get knowledgeable from good, reputable sources about all the ingredients. This will expand your adventure of making herbal body care products from herbs your have grown in your garden.

MIXING AND BLENDING

The good news is, making herbal products does not take fancy equipment. Most items can be found in an ordinary kitchen. To prevent cross contamination, consider using supplies that are set aside just for making your herbal spa recipes. Glass and metal can be cleaned thoroughly, but things that cannot be sterilized or are electronic, like a coffee bean grinder, are better used for just grinding herbs and blends used for body care recipes.

When melting or warming ingredients to liquefy, be patient! Never expose natural ingredients to high heat, use low to medium heat until the consistency is reached. Turn off heat and work quickly before ingredients harden again.

Blender: for making poultices and pulps from vegetables. Use a glass blender for whipping lotions and oils.

Coffee grinder (electric): for grinding herbs into a fine powder. Does the job perfectly.

Double boiler: for distributing even heat to help prevent oils and waxes from overheating or burning.

Eye dropper or pipettes: used for accurate dropper measurement of essential oils. Herb and soap suppliers (see Resources section) have disposable droppers to avoid cross contamination of different oils.

Funnels: various sizes for pouring ingredients into bottles. A wide mouth canning funnel works well when packaging dried herbs into fabric sachet bags.

Glass mixing bowls: an assortment of sizes for different mixes. Glass is easy to clean off residue, oil, and waxes.

Grater: for grating beeswax and soap bars to create small, melt-able pieces. Also good for lemon and lime zest.

Measuring spoons and cups: various kinds. Use glass measuring cups for oils and liquids. Metal or plastic ones are fine for measuring dried herbs.

Mortar and pestle: for crushing flowers and seeds. Also useful for making vegetable pulps.

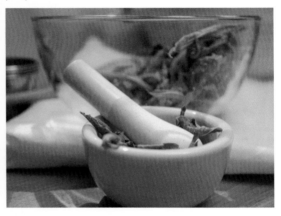

Sauce pans: glass or enamel in an array of sizes. Do not use aluminum, cast iron, copper or Teflon, as they can discolor herbs and affect quality of the mixes.

Stirring utensils: various kinds. Use wooden popsicle sticks, chopsticks and bamboo skewers when working with wax; they can be thrown away when done. Larger wooden spoons can be used to bruise herbs and push into liquids. A whisk comes in handy to help blend oils with other liquids.

STORAGE AND PACKAGING

For hand blended products: Store them in glass bottles and jars when possible and appropriate. Glass will help the herbs retain their precious oils. Bottles that are colored cobalt blue, green or amber are used to keep light from affecting the mixtures within. Tins can be used for salves and balms that stay solid at room temperature and for herb blends that have no moisture in them, such as dried tea mixes. Whenever possible, recycle glass canning jars and tins. Just be sure to clean and sterilize them well before use.

How to Sterilize Glass Jars

Wash the jars and scrub out any dust and debris with hot soapy water. If an oily residue is on the surface, swish glass with vodka. Rinse well and dry. Place the empty jars in a large pot and completely cover them with water. Bring the pot to a rolling boil over high heat and continue to boil for 15 minutes. Turn off the heat and allow to cool slightly. Remove jars from pan and air dry.

Packaging herbs for air travel: Use plastic bottles and zip-close bags and label everything. Plastic is not easily recyclable

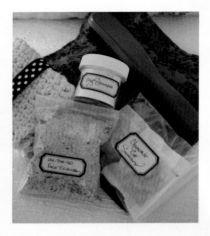

for second use because is hard to remove past debris and fragrance from the porous surface. Rinse new plastic containers with hot water and allow air dry completely before use.

Fabrics for sachets, bath bags and sleep pillows: These fabrics need to be 100 % cotton. Use unbleached natural muslin for anything that will be used in water, like bathing remedies and teas. Prewash fabric with fragrance-free washing soap to remove fabric sizing, chemicals and other odors.

QUICK TIPS FOR PREPARATION

- Avoid metal utensils – they can alter the color of waxes, oils and turn herbs black.

- Use glass or enamel heat-safe pans for simmering and melting.

- Never cook on high heat; raise heat slowly to warm or melt as needed. The smell of burnt waxes and herbs is not a good thing. And use caution when warming oils that may ignite.

- Always thoroughly clean, rinse and sterilize jars that are used for preparation and storage.

- To remove oil residue from glass: wipe or swish with vodka and rinse with scalding water.

- Use distilled or spring water in all preparations, not tap water that may have residue or sediment.

- Store in the proper size of jar. Use just enough to hold the amount without a lot of headspace.

- Carefully label everything. Herbs oils, salts and many ingredients look the same in a jar.

- Store finished products in a cool, dark place or as noted. Use immediately as needed.

- The fridge can be a good place to keep readymade products, just label them so they do not get accidently mistaken for something edible.

- Always be patient and mix, oil, waxes and waters together slowly to help them incorporate well.

Safety

Spa treatments use oil, water and other slippery ingredients. When slathered on the body, the dripping remnants can make stepping out of a tub or soaking bin dangerous. Always have a towel or bath mat next to you before a treatment so you can immediately step onto a dry, safe surface. Saunas and warm soaks can cause blood pressure to drop and cause lightheadedness upon standing. Rise slowly from any treatment, wait to feel clear-headed before walking. Falling asleep in a tub of deep, warm water can risk drowning; consider setting a timer to wake you after a half-hour of soaking.

THE RECIPES

Let's get started! Pick your inspiration
from the 11 themes below. The recipes,
DIY projects and tips will guide you
along through your spa experience.

■ ■ ■

GET STEAMY

TEA TIME

DOWN TO YOUR SOLES

A MANLY HERBAL

THE TOP-TO-BOTTOM SCRUB EXPERIENCE

JET LAG

MINT TO BE

FRAGRANT THERAPY

IN YOUR FACE

MIDSUMMER'S EVE CELEBRATION

WINTER SOLSTICE

GET STEAMY

Imagine the end of a long day, when rainy or cold weather feels like it has settled into every fiber of your body. You just want go home, relax, and chase away the chill. Create your own steam spa with a soothing cloud of fragrant herbs to surround you. I'm talking aromatherapy here.

Certain plants quickly release oils when exposed to heat. It is why on a hot summer day we are overcome (in a good way) by the fragrance of aromatic plants in the garden. They are naturally releasing their essential oils. When the body is exposed to warmth, it opens pores and allows the skin to easily accept the environment it is in. Combining herbs with hot steaming water or moist heat from a sauna is an experience that opens skin to take in all the natural benefits of the plants.

Heating up

In a sauna. Sauna, whether by water or by dry or humid air, is based on the principle of heating skin to a point of perspiration to release toxins and provide muscle relaxation. Blood flow is also directed to

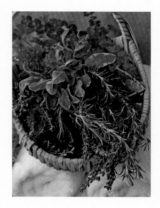

the skin, causing it to flush. In a sauna environment, the addition of fragrant herbs takes that physical reaction to a greater level. In a sauna, hang a muslin bag or place a small bowl filled with dried herbs to release as the air heats up.

No sauna? Do this instead. If you do not have access to an actual sauna, create your own sauna-like atmosphere in a bathroom. Use a small bathroom to easily capture heat and steam. Prepare the space, close windows and doors, roll up a towel to cover the crack along the bottom of the door and anywhere else heat will escape. Gather bath towels, a washcloth, fresh water bottle, a comfortable stool or chair, and the herb preparations. Give yourself at least 20 minutes to relax in the warmth.

Bath tub method:

Plug the drain and turn on hot water only. Run the water until the tub is about half full and the room begins to steam up. Add the herbs to the water and allow them to float across the surface. Sit comfortably next to the tub, relax and inhale the fragrant steam.

Shower method:

Hang a bundle of fresh herbs or dried sachets in the shower on a hook away from the spray of water but close enough to heat up.

Turn on hot water in the shower and run for about 10 to 15 minutes until the room is completely fogged with steam. Sit down and relax.

■ Herb Steam Bundles

Energy

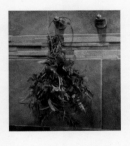

- Bundle 3 fresh-cut rosemary branches (approximately 10 to 12 inches long) and 3 fresh-cut peppermint stems together. Float in bath water or hang in the shower stall.

Relaxing

- Place 1 cup of fresh or dried lavender buds and 1 cup fresh or dried rose petals in a muslin bag to hang in the shower or float loose in bath water.

Healing

- Thinly slice about 2 tablespoons of fresh ginger, combine with 1 cup of fresh eucalyptus leaves, and place in muslin bag to hang in the shower or float loose in bath water.

Note: Heat is one of the more volatile ways to expose herbal power to skin and should be used with caution. Start with small amounts of herb and allow them to permeate the air. The heat is preparing your body to take in the herbal properties as it opens pores. The warmth also makes the herbs react and release their properties quickly, so keep in mind that a little goes a long way. Use extreme caution around the hot water to avoid burns.

Lavender Heat Pillow

This comfortable pillow can be draped over the neck and shoulders and is perfect to bring along if you are going into a public sauna. As the environment and your body heats up, the rice becomes humid and fragrant lavender aroma will be released in your personal space.

1 cup dried lavender buds
4 cups uncooked white rice
14 x 24-inch cotton hand towel or 100% cotton fabric, prewashed

What to do:

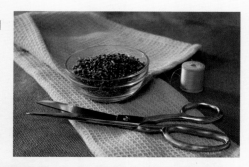

- Mix the rice and lavender buds together in a bowl and set aside.
- Fold the fabric in half (right sides together) and stitch along one end and the length opposite the fold. Turn right side out and press.
- Fill the open end with the lavender-rice mixture. Stitch closed.

For general use as a hot pack on sore muscles or across the back of the neck as a headache soother:

Heat in the microwave for approximately one minute or until warm, not burning to skin. The rice stays warm and the lavender will release its aromatic, healing fragrances. Can be used repeatedly.

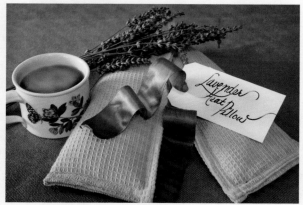

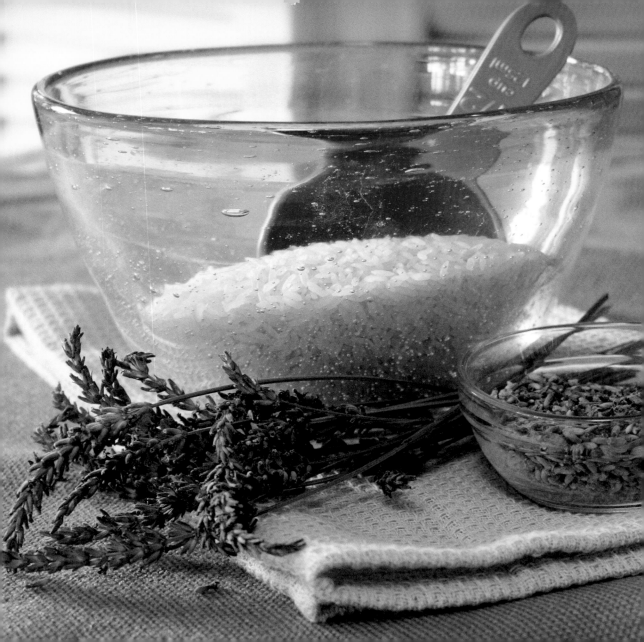

FACIAL STEAMS

Warm humidity on the skin is one of the easiest gentle cleansing rituals you can give your face. The delicate tissues of the skin are soothed as the steam rises. There is no harsh scrubbing or rubbing needed as the warmth increases perspiration and stimulates blood circulation. Perspiration is the body's natural cooling system and is just a release of water mixed with impurities. A gentle splash of water after a steam and those impurities are washed away.

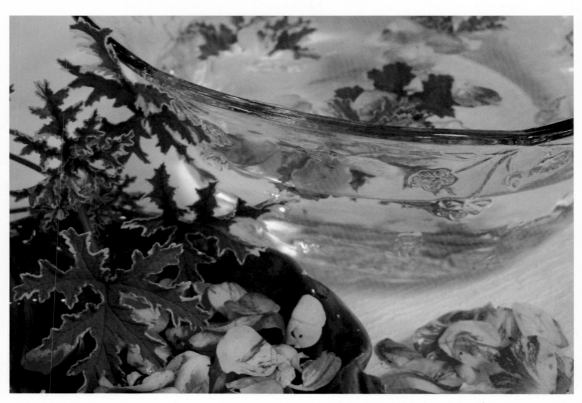

■ Mini Steam Sauna for the Face

Large glass bowl or small sink with stopper.
Large bath towel
Hot water
Herbs (see best choices for face steaming, below)
Fresh, cool water or optional lemon verbena water (see recipe below)

What to do:

- Pull hair away from face and gently wash skin, with a simple clean water rinse, unless skin has heavy makeup. Pat dry with a towel but leave skin dewy with some moisture.

- Place a handful of fresh, clean herbs in a glass bowl. Pour boiling water over them (about 3 cups) and allow to steep for about 5 minutes.

- Make a tent to capture the steam by covering head and shoulders with a large towel. Hold your head 12 inches away from steaming water and close your eyes. Take a few deeps breaths to inhale the fragrance of the herbs. Steam skin for 5 to 10 minutes.

- Remove towel drape and splash skin with cool water or wipe gently with cotton balls soaked in lemon verbena water (recipe below).

Herbs for Facial Steams

You may choose one herb or use in combination with others listed within the same category.

To boost circulation: rosemary, thyme

To soothe: chamomile, lavender, lemon balm, rose petals

For oily skin: calendula, rose geranium, sage

For dry and sensitive skin: borage, parsley, lavender

For mature skin: dandelion, lemon verbena, calendula, rose petals

■ Lemon Verbena Splash

1 cup loosely packed fresh lemon verbena leaves
¾ cup vodka

10 drops lemon verbena essential oil
1 cup distilled water

What to do:

■ Place fresh leaves into a sterilized glass jar. Pour vodka to completely cover the leaves.

■ Bruise the leaves with a wooden spoon or pestle. Add essential oil drops and cover tightly.

■ Allow to infuse for up to 2 weeks in a cool, dark place. Shake the jar every few days.

■ When mix smells heavy of lemon verbena, strain through a filter or cheesecloth to remove the leaves from the vodka.

■ Add distilled water, shake thoroughly.

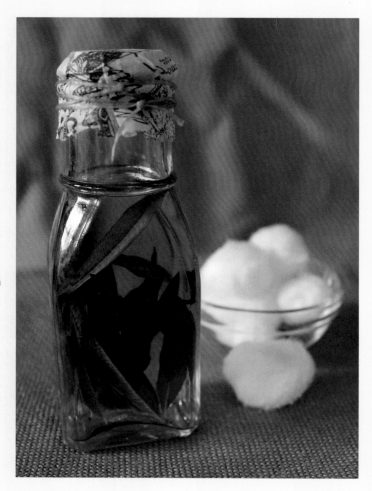

THE RITUAL OF BATHING

Do you need to take an adult timeout? Rediscover the art of bathing. Shut down the electronic devices, they simply don't do well when dropped near water! Surround yourself with things to unwind and create an escape. Bathing should be a sensual experience. The warmth of the water enveloping you can transport your mind and body through an herbal nurturing journey. It is vital to make time for this spa experience. Define the ritual and have supplies in a basket that are ready for you. I assure you, an hour out of a busy schedule is worth it.

■ ■ ■

Gather supplies:

Candles	Washcloths
Music	Towels
Bath pillow	Handmade spa treatments

Herbs in the bath can be healing, energizing and moisturizing, depending on the varieties you choose. As you use them you will discover more about their healing qualities and you can create your own custom blends.

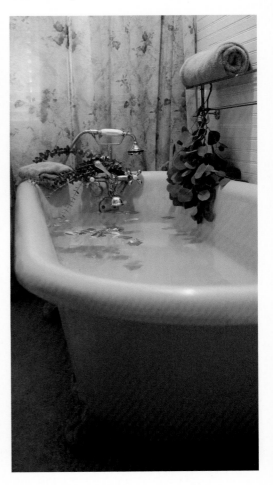

■ Basic Bath Brew

This is an easy way to add herb qualities to bathwater without a lot of preparation.

2 cups fresh herbs

1 quart water

A few drops essential oil
(optional)

What to do:

■ In a glass saucepan, bring water to boil. Remove pan from heat. Add herbs and allow to steep for at least 15 minutes.

■ Strain the herbs out. If desired, add a few drops of the same herb's essential oil to enhance the infusion.

■ Pour the herb water into a warm bath. Soak in the bath for at least 15 to 20 minutes to get the full effects of the herb.

■ Microwave option: heat water in a glass microwave-safe bowl for 2 minutes or until water is just starting to boil. Remove from microwave and add fresh herbs. Push the herbs in the water until they are completely covered and allow to sit for 15 minutes. Finish with essential oil as noted above.

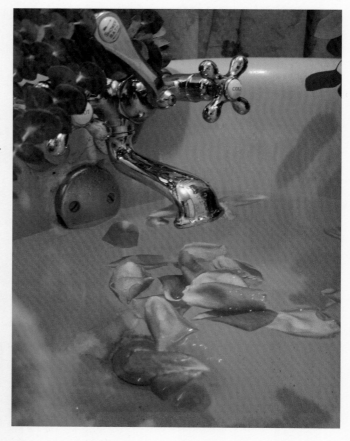

Bathing Herbs

Relaxing: chamomile, hops, lavender

Stimulating: basil, eucalyptus, lemon balm, mint, rosemary, sage, thyme

Healing: calendula, lavender, lemon verbena, parsley, spearmint

■ Inspiration Bath

Need to get some creativity flowing? This bath is especially effective the night before a stressful event or work project. The blend of essential oils works together to create a mental sense of wellbeing, while calendula flowers in the water nourish the skin. It is best to do right before bed and with a full night's sleep ahead. (See next page for information about essential oils.)

1 cup tightly packed fresh or dried calendula petals
6 drops lavender essential oil
6 drops rose essential oil

What to do:

- Place the blossoms directly in the bath or in a muslin sachet. Add the essential oils under running water to disburse them.

- Soak for 20 minutes in a quiet, relaxing atmosphere.

- For a morning treat: Upon waking, place 2 drops of peppermint essential oil and 2 drops of rosemary essential oil on a washcloth. Hold the cloth near your face and nose, inhale deeply and breathe out slowly. Repeat a few times. Add water to saturate the washcloth, wring out and use to wipe neck, shoulders and arms.

Things to Know About Essential Oils

When you walk into a garden on a warm summer afternoon and inhale the aroma of blooming lavender, you are smelling the essential oils being released by the heat of the sun. The natural flavoring used in mint chewing gum is from the essential oil from mint plants. Brush your hand along the stem of rosemary – that fragrance is from nature's chemicals being released on your fingers. Numerous compounds make up oils within the plants and give them fragrance, flavor and healing qualities. Bottled essential oils are literally the extracted essence of a plant and will have the most concentrated characteristics of plants.

Essential oils used in herbal treatments capture the true quality of herbs and will enhance recipes when used in addition to the natural plant. If there is an herb you can't grow or do not have available in the garden, typically the oil can be used to replace it.

Essential oil production itself is not something most herb gardeners will do at home. Plants do not always give up their essence readily and need to be distilled by water and/or steam methods. Plus, it can take pounds of high quality plant material to get a few precious drops.

When purchasing oils, how do you know if it is real *essential* oil? Essential oils are the pure form of the plant. These are not "perfume oil" or "aromatherapy oil." Because labeling is not regulated and can be ambiguous, here are some things to be alert to:

The label. Reputable companies will list the actual botanical name of the plant it was extracted from. Avoid an oil that has other ingredients added; it is common to adulterate oils with synthetic versions of fragrance or with an unscented base oil.

The price. This is a big factor. Not all oils are the same price because of the process to make them. For example, it takes 5 tons of rose petals to obtain only 2 pounds of essential oil, making pure rose oil one of the pricier ones on the market. Plants that produce abundant oil and take less plant material to extract from, like mint, are usually less expensive. It all comes down to what the plant will yield. If a supplier lists all oils with the same size bottles and price, be wary. My best advice is to purchase from trusted sources who sell oils for body care.

Use caution! Plant essence oils are powerful and concentrated. The chemical components of most oils are intense and may harm the skin if used straight from the bottle. Keep out of reach of children, avoid use near eyes or mucus membranes, and do not take internally. To use safely, count out drops in correct amounts and mix properly with other ingredients.

To dilute an essential oil for general use: Blend 5 to 10 drops of essential oil per ounce of a neutral carrier oil such as jojoba or sweet almond oil.

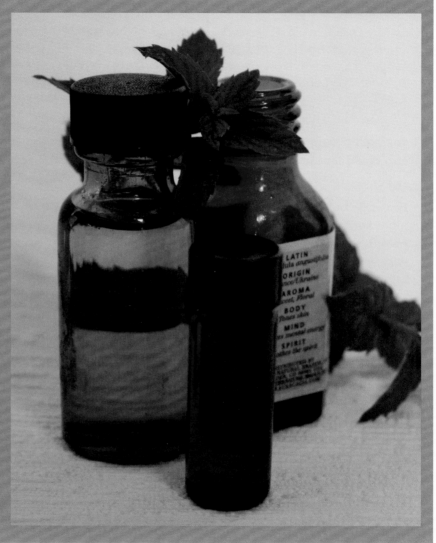

■ Oatmeal Soak

Oats have been used for centuries as a remedy to heal skin from rashes, bug bites, and after a tangle with poison ivy. It relieves itch and irritation, and it has cleansing qualities from the saponins present in the plant. Studies show that the phenols in the oats actually have antioxidant and anti-inflammatory properties. All those qualities are contained in good old-fashioned oatmeal, the kind you cook for breakfast. So when you combine oatmeal with herbs chosen for their special properties, you create a rich mix that will cleanse and heal.

1 cup rolled oats
1 cup dried lemon verbena leaves

1 cup dried lavender buds
1 cup dried rosebuds and petals

What to do:

■ In a large bowl, gently mix all of the ingredients together. Use your hands to help the rose and lemon verbena combine with the smaller ingredients.

■ Place the mix in muslin bags and store for use at any time. This blend can also be ground to a fine powder that disperses easily in water.

To use:

■ Hang the bag from the tub faucet as the bath is filling up. When the water is turned off, float the herb bag in the water. To gain the full benefits, allow for a bath time of at least 15 minutes or longer.

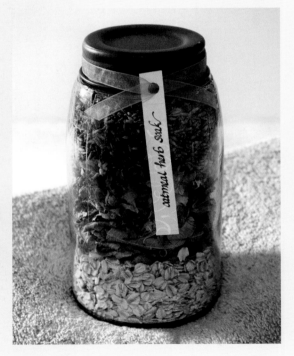

Is it Just Oatmeal?

Rolled, old-fashioned, quick cooking, steel-cut, colloidal? You can find these all on store shelves, and yes, they are all made from oats (*Avena sativa*). The difference is how they are processed. Rolled oats, sometimes called old-fashioned, are oat grain kernels steamed and flattened into flakes. Quick or instant are oat flakes rolled thinner to cook faster. Steel-cut is oat kernels cut (not rolled) into smaller pieces. Colloidal oatmeal is the oats ground into an extremely fine powder.

For cosmetic and spa treatments, the only two types you need to know are rolled and colloidal. Rolled, whole organic oats mix well with bulky herbs and are used in bath blends and body scrubs. The powdered version, colloidal oatmeal, is widely used in the cosmetic industry for a milky texture that disperses the oats to coat and moisturize skin as you soak in a tub of water.

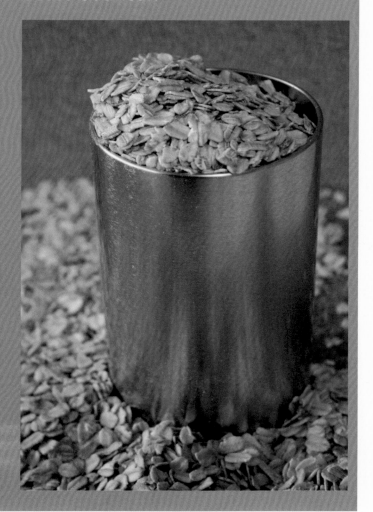

TEA TIME

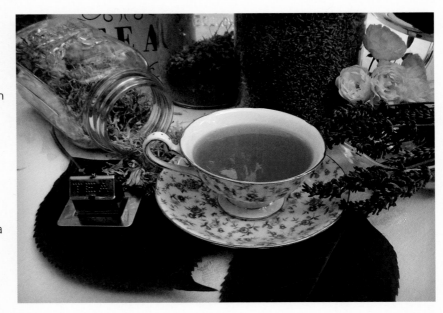

For me, just saying the words "tea time" evokes sweet memories of an afternoon with a fresh brewed cup of tea in the Palm Court at the Ritz in London. Ahhh, tea: It can be a ritual, an herb, a beverage – or all three. Technically, tea is the plant *Camellia sinensis*. Varieties of true tea plants are not cultivated in many home gardens. The leaves of these sub-tropical evergreen shrubs are processed to create different selections of tea, like black or oolong. Tea's rich history is filled with scandals, political and personal, and even a declaration of independence. Today, tea has evolved into a mind-boggling palette of blends; it is sold in many forms, from rich, black C. sinensis to herbal infusions combining an array of plants. In its simplest definition, the basic term "tea" refers to plant parts steeped in warm water to create a flavored beverage.

Create your own elegant tea-time tradition with a sensual touch. This spa experience takes tea inside and out of the body, using herbs from your garden to make tub teas for bathing and custom blends for sipping.

Tub Tea

Tub teas are really just oversized tea bags that turn bathwater into an herbal delight. The best method is to place dried herbs in fabric sachets or press and seal oversized tea bags (see resource section). Use single herbs per bag, mix and match as you please, depending on your mood. Make up a bunch of these ahead of time and store individual varieties in large glass jars.

How to package tub teas:

Packaging herb mixes for bathing in sachet bags will prevent clogged drains and an unpleasant mess of herbs sticking to your skin as you emerge from the tub. Place single varieties of dried herbs in individual, oversized versions of a typical tea bag. The bags can be purchased from health food stores and herbal suppliers…or you can make your own with the how-to on the next page.

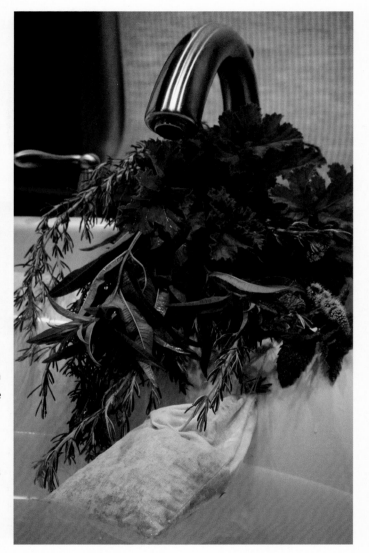

■ Make-Your-Own Oversized Tea Bags

An 8 x 15-inch piece of washed cotton muslin,
    (100% cotton fabric with no dyes that will bleed into the water)
Dried herbs

What to do:

- Cut all the fabric edges around with pinking shears. Fold fabric in half lengthwise.

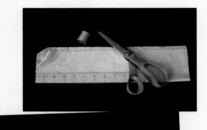

- Use dressmaker's chalk or a washable marker and mark the fabric in thirds.

- Machine stitch ¼-inch away on each side of the vertical lines and along both vertical edges.

- Fill each pocket with your chosen tub tea herb. Stitch the entire row across the top, ¼-inch away from top.

- Cut along vertical lines with pinking shears to separate individual bags.

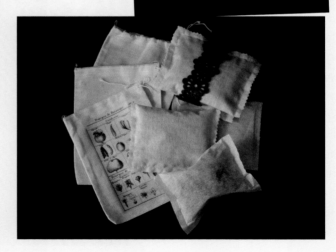

A real tea bath

Camellia sinensis on the skin has been the subject of recent studies by the cosmetic industry. Benefits attributed to the topical use of green tea include anti-aging, anti-inflammatory, and healing on irritated skin. Green tea is the unfermented leaves of *C. sinensis*, and one of the least processed methods of the leaves. Mild blends of green tea leaves mixed with herbs make a good addition to bathing. Toss two regular-sized tea bags in your bath water and reap the fragrant, healing rewards.

■ Lavender Green Tub Tea

What to do:
- In a large tub tea sachet, combine 1 tablespoon organic loose green tea and 4 tablespoons dried lavender buds.

To Use:
- Add lavender green tub tea bag to bath as warm water is filling the tub to allow tea to begin to disperse into the water. Soak in the herbal tea water for at least 15 minutes to reap full benefits.

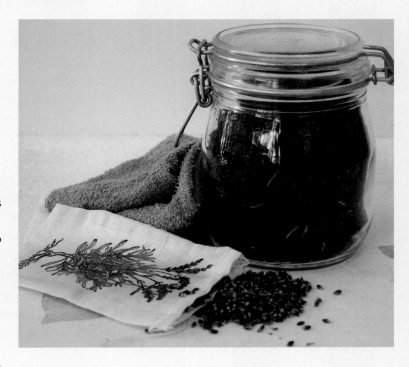

How to make a fresh pot of herb tea:

Boil water in a teakettle. Transfer boiling water into a warmed glass or ceramic teapot. Add a handful of fresh herbs and allow to steep for at least 10 minutes, longer for stronger tea.

Most herbal blends do not reach a deep dark color; they will remain light amber or green. Gauge your herbal brew by taste rather than by color. Dried herbs are more concentrated, so use less quantity than fresh leaves. A rule of thumb is 1 teaspoon of dried herbs or 3 teaspoons of fresh herbs to 1 cup of water.

Herbal tea recipe blends:

Many blends or single teas can be made with plants from the garden. Store your custom blends in sealed jars or tins. Based on the type of taste you want, mix two or three varieties of herbs together to balance the flavor.

Here are some recipes to try. Mix these blends and store in lidded glass jars.

To use: 1 teaspoon of loose dry herbs (or 3 teaspoons of fresh herbs) per cup of hot water.

Sweet, Minty and Soothing
½ cup dried lavender buds
1 cup dried spearmint
½ cup dried peppermint

A Tangy Touch of Citrus
¼ cup of dried citrus peel, cut into ¼ inch pieces (lemon, orange or a mix)
1 cup rose hips, lightly crushed
½ cup dried lemon balm

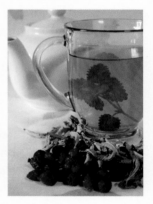

A Floral Blend
½ cup rose petals
½ cup lavender buds
¼ cup chamomile flowers

Herbs mixed with traditional *Camellia sinensis:*

Create your own flavorful mixtures from purchased bulk teas. Mix a single herb with bulk tea such as Darjeeling, green or Earl Grey to create unique blends. Your homegrown herb (dried) will enhance the tea with flavor and fragrance.

The basic recipe to create blends with traditional tea is 4 parts tea to 1 part dried herb. Experiment with the flavor intensity and add more herbs to enhance or more tea to tone down.

Some combinations to try:

English lavender buds with Earl Grey
Spearmint with green tea
Lemon Balm with Oolong
Rose petals with Darjeeling
Chamomile flowers with white tea

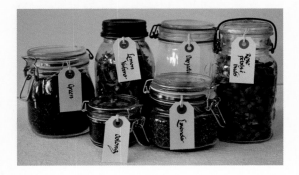

Fresh Herbal Sun Tea

Fill a gallon glass jar halfway with fresh, clean herb leaves, buds or flowers. Cover herbs with cold water, until jar is full. Place in the sun and allow to steep for 4 to 6 hours. Strain out herbs before serving.

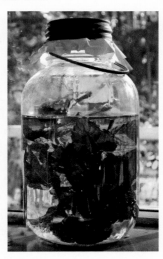

Loose Tea and Herb Iced Tea

If you have a favorite type of tea such as green or Darjeeling, use 7 regular-sized tea bags to 1 cup of fresh herb leaves. Steep in the sun following the above recipe. Remove the tea bags and herbs before serving. Serve with herbal ice cubes for extra flavor (see how-to under preserving, page 80).

DOWN TO YOUR SOLES

In ancient Greece, the philosopher Diogenes soaked his feet in aromatic plants, reasoning that it was wasteful to use them on one's head where the scent rose into the air to benefit only the birds. By using it on his feet, he could bathe his whole body and senses in the rising fragrance.

The beginning of pure relaxation starts at the bottom. Feet take the weight of the world; to create a pampering experience for them is one of the simplest, indulgent spa techniques. Once you have all the supplies, the setup is quick and can almost be done anywhere, even in the garden.

All you need is a bowl or low-sided tub large enough to fit both feet comfortably. Take a moment to prepare everything before you step into the water. Place all of your needed items in a basket within reach. Choose a comfortable chair with a pillow for back support and be able to place feet firmly in the bowl. Place the bowl on a towel, lay another towel next to it to wrap your feet in after the foot treatment.

A rocky massage

Give yourself a foot massage by placing a layer of polished, smooth stones in the bottom of the bowl before adding water. Slowly work the balls of your feet over the stones repeatedly while soaking, for enchanting massage benefits.

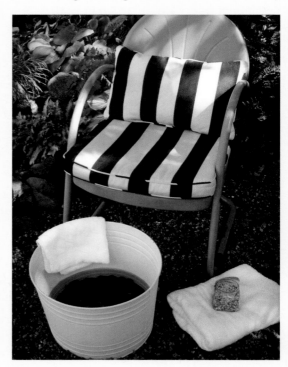

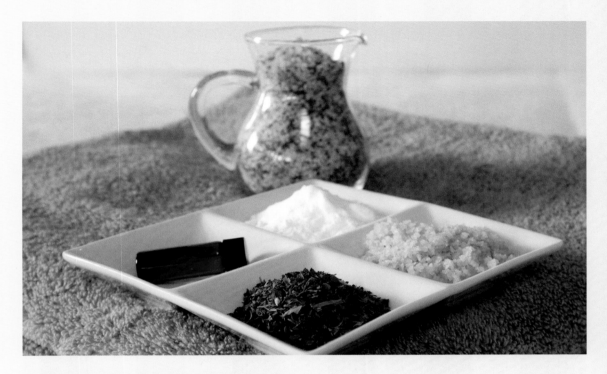

▪ Peppermint Foot Soak

1 cup coarse sea salt

½ cup baking soda

½ cup dried peppermint, crushed

2 drops peppermint essential oil (optional)

What to do:

- Combine all ingredients well and store in a lidded glass jar. For a finer blend that will disperse in water easier, you may grind all of the ingredients together.

- Place mix in a bowl or small tub of warm water. Soak feet for a minimum of 15 minutes to capture the full benefits.

Which Salt is the Right Salt?
(coarse, fine, rock, table, Epsom, sea)

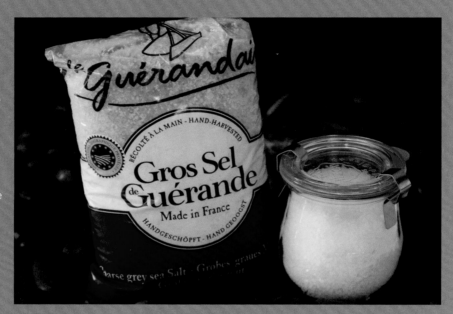

Let's take a quick look at salt. Common salt is sodium chloride. Coarse and fine both describe how salts are ground. Rock salt is larger pieces of sodium chloride and table salt is finely ground for cooking. Typically, table salt is heavily processed and treated with additives to keep it free-flowing. Epsom salt is named after a salt spring in England. It is not actually salt, but a naturally occurring compound of magnesium and sulfate. Epsom salt is readily absorbed by skin and has numerous health benefits. The magnesium reduces inflammation and helps muscles relax and function better. The sulfate helps absorption of nutrients and also flushes toxins from the body. Sea salt is produced by the evaporation of seawater and depending on the source contains trace natural minerals. It is most often used for bathing and scrubs because of its mineral compound and natural harvesting process. For spa treatments and skin care regimens, use sea salt and Epsom salt.

Cooling Herbal Foot Powder

1 tablespoon dried lemon thyme leaves,
  finely ground
1 teaspoon dried peppermint leaves,
  finely ground
1 teaspoon dried parsley leaves

⅓ cup cornstarch
2 tablespoons baking soda
1 to 2 drops peppermint or
lemon essential oil (optional)

What to do:

■ Mix dry ingredients well and, if desired, add the essential oil. Place in a zip-close bag or sealed jar and shake well. Grind ingredients together if needed to make the mix finer.

■ Store in glass jar with shaker lid.

To use:

■ Sprinkle the powder on clean, dry feet and work into skin with a gentle massage motion.

■ Can also be used to freshen the inside of shoes.

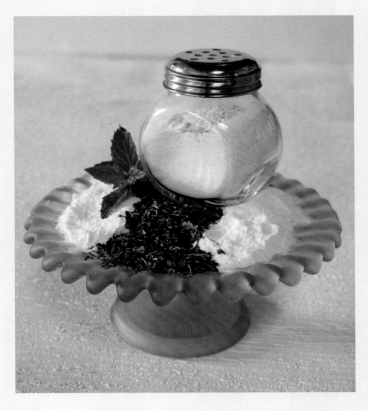

▪ Sweet Feet Sugar Scrub

1 cup organic raw sugar
Approximately ¼ cup fresh
   spearmint leaves, cut into small pieces
Approximately ¼ cup fresh
   rosemary leaves

⅓ cup grapeseed oil
1 Vitamin E capsule
Lime zest to add fragrance and
enhance color (optional)

What to do:

- In a small, wide-mouth canning jar, add about an inch of sugar. Add a layer of spearmint; pour enough sugar to cover leaves. Place a layer of rosemary leaves, cover with sugar, then alternate layers of herbs and sugar until the jar is full.

- Use immediately, or for a richer result, cover jar and allow to sit for 5 to 7 days. The sugar will be highly fragrant from absorbing the essential oils from the leaves.

To use:

- Add grapeseed oil to the herb sugar jar. Pierce the Vitamin E capsule and squeeze into mix. Add the lime zest, if desired. Mix and let sit for about 5 minutes to allow the oil to soak into the sugar.

- Prepare a tub of fresh, warm water and set aside. Lay out a towel on the ground. Massage a generous scoop of the sugar scrub to clean bare feet for about 5 minutes per foot. Gently massage and work through toes and all over the bottom of the feet. Scrub more vigorously on rough skin at the heels.

- Rinse and allow feet to rest in the tub of water for another 5 minutes.

- Place feet on the towel and wrap around to bundle up both feet and hold in warmth. Relax and enjoy.

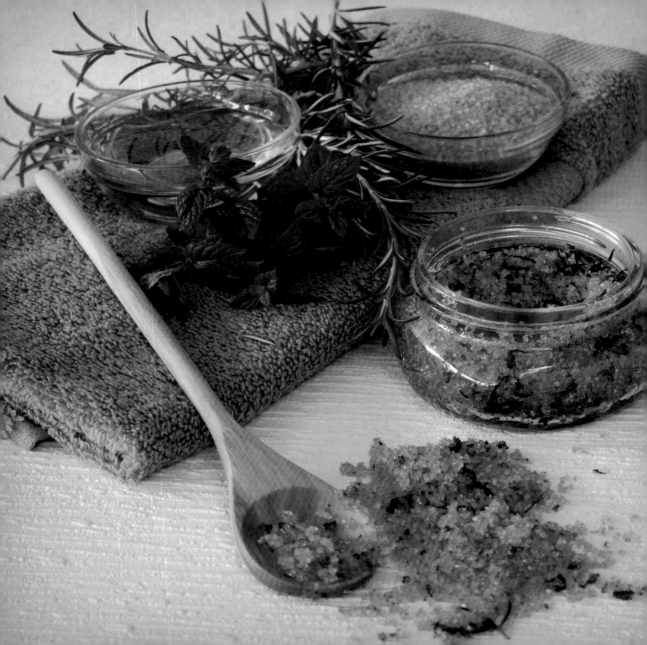

A MANLY HERBAL

The fragrances of basil, rosemary and thyme are rich with notes of camphor, pepper, pine and clove. There are no flowery, perfumed undertones. It's all about a deep timbre of aroma – not delicate flowers. A woman's sense of smell is more sensitive than a man's; perhaps it is why men's cosmetics have stronger, earthy aromas. Intense infusions of herbs combined with nourishing oils and ingredients are targeted to a man's senses and skin needs.

■ Beard and Face Cleanser

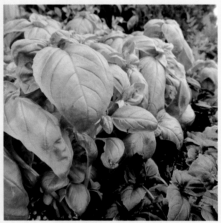

The skin on a man's face takes a beating from constant shaving. Even with facial hair, the skin underneath is experiencing constant change from skin cells and oil. Treat with care by using herbs infused in a natural olive oil-based soap. Use this for a daily cleanse or just before a sauna or steam soak.

1 cup pure Castile liquid soap
½ cup basil infusion

Basil Infusion:

■ Bring 1 cup of water to a boil in a glass sauce pan. Remove the pan from heat and add 3 to 5 fresh basil leaves. Cover and allow to steep for 15 minutes. Remove and discard the basil leaves from the water by filtering through cheesecloth. Pour Castile liquid soap into a sterilized glass jar, add the basil infusion, and shake well to mix.

To use:

■ Splash face with warm water. Lather cleanser on face with a gentle massage through facial hair. Rinse with cool water. Pat skin dry.

▪ Wisdom Toner and Aftershave

Sage is the herb of wisdom. Ancient herbalists praised it for improving brain function, and for memory and dementia. The Romans had a saying,, "Cur morietur homo, cui salvia crescuit in horto?" (How can a man die who has sage growing in his garden?) Historical usage has even made sage a synonym for the word "wise".

For this toner and aftershave, I combine sage with lavender and witch hazel. The witch hazel lends its cleansing and pore tightening properties to the mix.

½ cup fresh sage leaves, rinsed
4 tablespoons dried lavender flowers

½ cup witch hazel extract, homemade or purchased true witch hazel extract (see recipe on the following page)

What to do:

- In a clean glass jar, add the sage leaves and lavender. Pour witch hazel over the leaves and slightly crush inside the jar with a wooden spoon or pestle.

- Place a lid on the jar tightly and shake well. Allow to steep for one week. Shake the jar daily to mix. Strain thoroughly. This might take more than one filtering through cheesecloth to remove all of the residue.

- Pour into a clean bottle and store in a cool location. Shake well before each use. If reserved witch hazel extract is used, can be stored for up to 6 months.

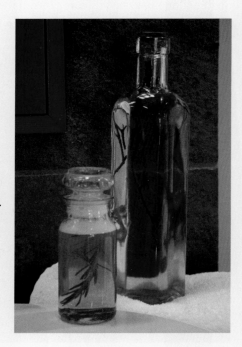

WITCH HAZEL EXTRACT

Sometimes a product is easier to purchase than make, and witch hazel extract is one of them. But…to further your herbal adventure, it is possible to make your own witch hazel if you have *Hamamelis virginiana* growing in your garden.

Prune a handful of fresh twigs from the shrub just after the plant has flowered. Strip off any leaves or flower remnants and cut the twigs into small pieces. Place the twigs in a glass saucepan and cover with distilled water. Use just enough water to cover the twigs completely (approximately 2 to 3 cups of water). Bring mix to a boil. Reduce heat, cover and simmer for 30 minutes. Allow to cool to room temperature and strain out bark from the water with cheesecloth. Use this fresh brew within a week. To give the infusion a longer shelf life, preserve by adding 1 cup of vodka.

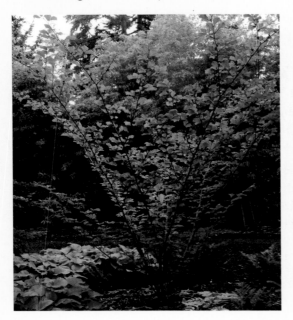

The bark of witch hazel *Hamamelis virginiana* is covered with transverse lenticels (breathing pores), which are similar to small wounds on human skin. In history, herbalists used the plant to heal wounds it resembled. Still popular today, a tincture of the shrubby witch hazel from leaves and bark is available at natural foods markets and health food stores. The plant has cleansing and astringent qualities.

For spa treatments, use a true witch hazel extract with lower alcohol content. The typical distilled witch hazel found in drugstores can contain up to 14% alcohol, which can be harsh on skin.

▪ Hand and Nail Butter

Tension can elicit pain in any part of the body, but sometimes a massage to one area can release tension in another. If arms and shoulders are tense, the simplicity of a hand massage begins to soothe and release. Hand massage techniques can be done anywhere to help ease stress, especially after working outside or on a computer all day. This recipe is rich in natural waxes and oils to saturate the skin in herbal goodness. This is great as a fingernail and cuticle treatment. For an intensive overnight treatment, use butter on the hands and feet, and wear socks and gloves to help seal in moisture.

2 tablespoons cocoa butter

2 tablespoons beeswax

4 tablespoons grapeseed oil

8 drops lavender essential oil

4 drops lemon essential oil

3 drops rose geranium essential oil

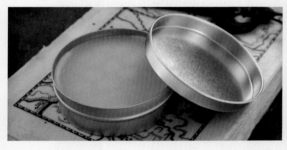

What to do:

- In a small saucepan, slowly melt cocoa butter and beeswax. Stir until well blended together and liquefied. Add grapeseed oil, stir well and remove from heat. Continue stirring until almost cooled down.

- Add the essential oils, stir well and pour into jar. The mixture will harden slightly to a smooth, buttery texture. Use this within 3 months for best freshness.

- **Give this hand massage to a partner or friend:** Apply a small amount of hand and nail butter to your friend's hand. Support one hand with your fingers and begin to stroke the ends of the fingers, working each finger gently along the joints and fingers. Work your way up to the wrist with gentle motions, spreading the herbal lotion as you go. Then sandwich their hand between your own hands and draw away very slowly and deliberately. Repeat several times before letting go completely. Repeat the motions on the other hand.

THE TOP-TO-BOTTOM SCRUB EXPERIENCE

Exfoliate! Invigorate! Revive! Body scrubs filled with herbs and abrasive materials gently massaged into the skin – these are a spa experience all their own. Blood circulates close to the skin, which pinks up with warmth as dead skin cells and impurities wash away. From the soles of the feet to the top of your head, spa treatments with texture help skin to feel renewed. Scrubs also help to flush toxins after healing from a cold or flu.

It is all about the formula and application: Blends with sea salt are good for oily skin; sugar is better for normal to dry skin; cornmeal is used for gentle facials, leaving skin smooth and refreshed with natural vitamins and moisture.

Scrubs can be used vigorously to heal and smooth rough skin, or with a lighter motion on delicate tissues. Pressure of application is important. On the face, use gentle, circular scrubbing motions. From the neck down, scrub with more pressure, especially on areas with cellulite. This is really not a relaxing massage type of treatment; it is an energizer.

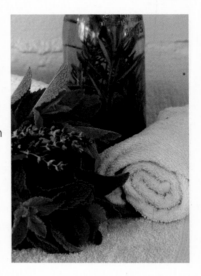

A full body scrub needs to take place in a shower or tub. Prepare your spa with fluffy towels, bright light, and upbeat music. Step in the shower first to rinse and dampen skin. Turn off the water and place a towel on the floor. The oil in the scrub may drip and cause a slippery surface, so use caution. Apply scrub, starting along the neck and using gentle motions, work your way down the body. Be kind while working with a scrub – skin should be nice and pink, not red or irritated. After application, rinse mixture from skin and gently pat skin dry with a soft towel. Follow a scrub treatment with a nourishing lotion to polish off and pamper your skin.

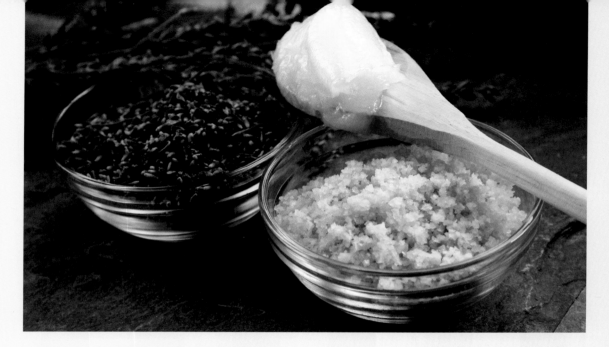

■ Lavender Spa Salt Glow

1 cup coarse gray sea salt
¾ cup coconut oil
6 drops lavender essential oil

2 tablespoons fresh or dried
   lavender buds

What to do:

■ Place all ingredients in a wide-mouth jar and mix well.

To use:

■ Dampen skin. With a generous amount of salt/oil mix, massage onto the skin with gentle circular motion. Use caution around scratched or irritated areas of skin. Rinse off with warm water.

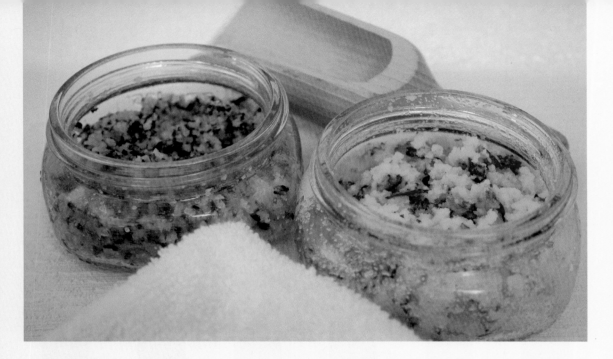

▪ Floral Sugar Scrub

2 cups sugar
1 cup coconut oil

1 Vitamin E capsule
½ cup fresh rose petals

What to do:

▪ Mix sugar, coconut oil and rose petals in a wide-mouth glass jar. Pierce the Vitamin E capsule and squeeze into the mix.

To use:

▪ Dampen skin. With a generous amount of floral scrub, massage onto the skin with gentle circular motion. Use caution around scratched or irritated areas of skin. Rinse off with warm water.

▪ A Homemade Spa Cloth

For the crocheter: Make this easy-to-do spa cloth. Made with 100% cotton yarn, the texture is just nubby enough to use with scrubs without being too abrasive. The cloth will measure approximately 12 x 12 inches when finished. Exact gauge is not necessary for this project.

1 ball of 100% cotton yarn, 4-ply, 2.5-ounce
Crochet hook, size H or 8

To make:

■ Chain 39 as the foundation row (see Resources section for more crochet information)

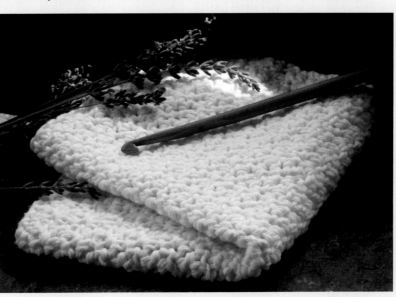

■ Row 1: single crochet in second chain from hook and in each chain until end.

■ Row 2: chain 1 and turn. Single crochet in first stitch, double crochet in next stitch. *single crochet in next stitch, double crochet in next stitch, repeat from * across.

■ Repeat row 2 for a total of 35 rows.

■ Row 36: single crochet in each stitch across, fasten off and weave in ends to finish.

▪ Après-Scrub Skin Oil

This is a light, simple oil that nourishes freshly scrubbed skin. Vanilla is a sensual fragrance that balances mood and relaxes.

1 cup jojoba oil
2 whole vanilla beans

What to do:

- Start with a sterilized glass bottle. Slice vanilla beans lengthwise, scrape out the center mush and place it in the bottle. Chop the beans into small pieces and add them to the bottle.

- Pour oil over the vanilla to cover completely. Place lid on the bottle and shake to mix well.

- Store in a cool, dark place for up to two months (shake every couple of weeks). When the vanilla aroma is intense, it is ready.

- Strain the oil through a mesh filter to remove bean remnants, and rebottle. If desired, add another whole vanilla bean to the finished bottle to add additional fragrance.

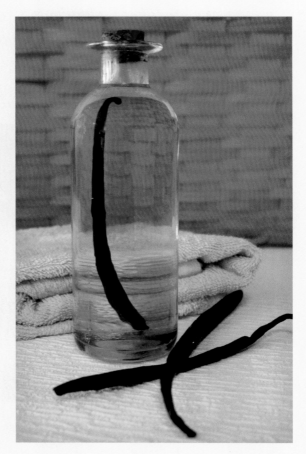

JET LAG

Long hours of travel sitting on a plane, train or car can zap your energy. Changes in elevation, weather, and culture all wreak havoc on the body and mind. Revive with on-the-go spa treatments packed for your next trip. Pack an herbal travel kit that is security friendly and doesn't take up too much space in your luggage. Herb

sachets for tub teas, dream pillows and soothing herbal treatments will help revive you while traveling.

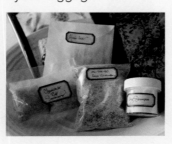

What to Pack:

Nighttime Mini-Spa for Sleep:
Chamomile tea bags for drinking
Tub tea sachets filled with lavender buds
Sleep pillow

After a day of travel, relax in a warm tub drinking a hot cup of tea and retire to fragrant herbs with a sleep pillow.

Sleep Pillows

These are sweet, small pillows filled with herbs. Tuck one into your hotel pillowcase for restful sleep while away from home. In aromatherapy practice, inhaling herbs help relax, calm or uplift and energize. These pillows draw on that aromatic power, based on the type of herbs used.

These not just haphazard mixes stuffed in fabric, but carefully chosen herbs and quantities that promote restful sleep. If there is an herb that transports your memory into a peaceful place, use it to mask the sterile odor of hotel rooms and guest linens.

The sleep pillows are stitched to be travel sized. Store in plastic zip-close bags. Remove pillow from plastic bag and tuck into pillowcase upon arrival to begin scenting the linens before going to bed.

Or, instead of a plastic bag, wrap your pajamas around the sleep pillow. When you're ready for bed at your destination, your pajamas will lightly scent the bedclothes.

▪ Sleep Pillows

Herb mix
2 cups dried lemon balm
1 cup dried hops

1 cup dried lavender buds
⅓ cup dried roses

What to do:

- Blend ingredients well and use to fill fabric pillows. Your sleep pillow may last for several months or years, based on the herbs used in the mix. *Option:* add just a single favorite herb with the hops.

To make:

- Cut two 8 x 8-inch squares from 100 % cotton fabric that has been prewashed to remove any odors. Wrong sides together, stitch closed on 3 sides. Turn right side out. Fill at the unstitched end with the herb mixture. Do not overfill, a few cups of mix should do. Stitch closed.

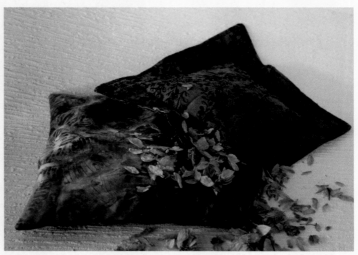

▪ Headache Pillow

If you have a tendency to get headaches due to airline cabin pressure or neck strain, there is an herb for that. Place this mix in a fabric pillow to create a headache relief pillow.

Herb mix:

Equal parts dried lavender flowers and lemon balm leaves.

DREAMY HERBS

Calendula petals: add calming restfulness with a citrus note.

Chamomile flowers: well-known for promoting sweet dreams. Use caution, if you have ragweed allergies. Chamomile is in the same plant family and may cause an allergic reaction.

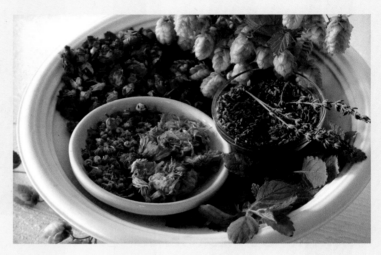

Hop cones: the most revered herb for promoting sleep. Some hop varieties are bitter while others are sweet. It is the common, sweet varieties used to induce sleep.

Lavender flowers: relaxing and calming, a more fragrant ingredient of a sleep pillow.

Lemon balm: highly valued to soothe depression, anxiety and insomnia.

Lemon verbena: with a rich lemon aroma known for a calming mood that does not necessarily bring deep sleep, but a relaxing sleep.

Rose petals: for comfort and warmth. The scent of roses promotes peacefulness when inhaled deeply. Reminiscent of a calming walk through a fragrant rose garden on a warm summer evening.

Herbs that will hold fragrance for a long time: Lavender, rose petals, lemon verbena.

Herbs that will dissipate after 6 months or less: hops, lemon balm, calendula, chamomile.

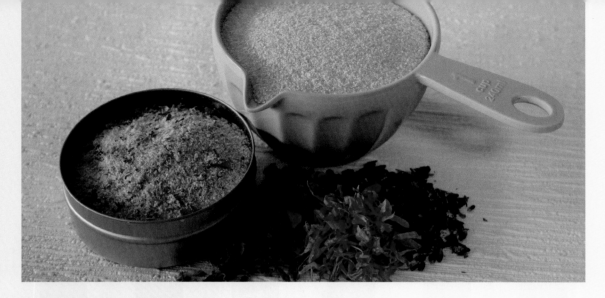

■ On-the-Go Face Scrub

Take this dry blend with you when you travel. At your destination, just add water or plain yogurt to create a nourishing skin treat that refreshes tired skin.

1 tablespoon dried rose petals

1 tablespoon dried lavender buds

1 tablespoon dried calendula petals

1 cup cornmeal

What to do:

- ■ Grind dried herbs together until powdered.
- ■ Add cornmeal and mix well.
- ■ Store in small plastic zip-close bags.

To use:

- ■ Rinse face, pat dry. Mix blend with just enough water or yogurt to form a paste. Gently massage paste over face and neck avoiding eye area. Rinse off and pat skin dry.

■ Chamomile Eye Soothers

Check your baggage (under your eyes) and ease dark circles and swelling with these tiny sachets.

Chamomile flowers   **Press-and-seal tea bags**

What to do:
- Fill tea bags with chamomile flowers and seal closed.

To use:
- Place tea bag in a small saucer. Pour 1 tablespoon of warm water over the bag to re-hydrate the flowers. Wait for the sachets to cool down. Gently squeeze excess water. Lie down, relax and apply to eyelids for 15 minutes.

■ Herbal Dry Shampoo

This dry shampoo gives an energizing refresh to the scalp after a long travel day.

⅓ cup cornstarch   **2 drops lemon essential oil**
3 drops lavender essential oil

What to do:
- Place cornstarch in a glass jar. Add the drops of essential oil. Cover the jar and shake well to allow the oils to permeate the cornstarch. For travel, place the mix in a small plastic jar or zip-close bag, and label.

To use:
- Sprinkle a small amount close to scalp. Massage scalp and work through hair with the tips of fingers. Allow to remain on hair for 5 minutes. Vigorously brush hair to disperse. You can also sprinkle the mix directly onto a hairbrush to work the powder through hair. The cornstarch will absorb oils while essential oils refresh the scalp and hair. If you are prone to oily hair, apply the dry shampoo before going to bed and leave in. Brush in the morning.

MINT TO BE

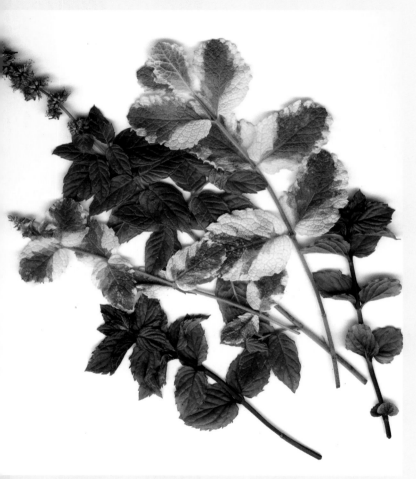

Refresh, stimulate, renew: all describe what mint will do for you. Mint is an all-natural essence with deep notes of camphor and just enough sweetness. The main constituent of mint is menthol. This unusual crystal-like substance causes a sensation of cold that is widely popular in the cosmetic industry for mouthwashes and toothpaste. The obvious attribute is its recognizable pungent fragrance, but its healing qualities are respectable too. It is a tonic and stimulant. Upon inhalation, it can energize the mind, uplift the mood and is reputed to be good for the nervous system. Let mint be your energizer.

▪ Scalp Tingle Mint Shampoo

A good morning wake-up! This tingly shampoo will smell great in the warmth of a shower, but also gets blood circulating in your brain.

1 cup loosely packed fresh mint
  leaves, whole
1 cup distilled water
1 cup pure liquid Castile soap
2 drops peppermint essential oil

What to do:

▪ Bring water to a boil in a glass
saucepan and remove from heat. Add
peppermint leaves and allow to steep
for a minimum of 15 minutes.

▪ Strain out the peppermint leaves, add
the essential oil, and then mix with
Castile soap.

▪ Shake well to mix and store in a plastic
bottle with a flip-top lid.

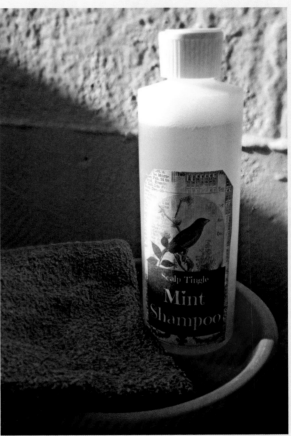

2 AT-WORK REVIVERS

■ Sweet vanilla-mint solid perfume

This can be tucked in the desk drawer at work. Rub a little on your wrists for an afternoon refresh.

2 tablespoons beeswax	**4 drops peppermint essential oil**
2 tablespoons sweet almond oil	**5 drops vanilla oil**

What to do:

■ Melt the beeswax until it is liquid. Add the sweet almond oil.

■ Allow to cool slightly and add peppermint and vanilla oil.

■ Stir well to mix to create a smooth texture.

■ Pour into a small tin or jar. Will harden upon cooling.

■ ■ ■

■ On-the-Go Minty Massage

Need a quick pick-me-up? Keep a stash of peppermint tea bags handy. Here's a light self-massage that uses mint's reviving fragrant qualities.

What to do:

■ Make a cup of strong peppermint-infused water by warming the tea bag in about 4 ounces of water. Dip your fingers in the warm water and massage your temples.

Temple massage technique:

■ This is a simple technique and when combined with mint is a quick way to boost energy and increase concentration. Use your middle and ring fingers, find the soft spot on your temples, which is between your eye and upper ear just along the hairline. Use gentle circles to massage the light, minty water into your skin. Apply gentle pressure and work in small circular motions, counting to ten. Take a few deep breaths and continue the circular massage. Dip fingers in water as needed. The massage will release tension while the mint takes action.

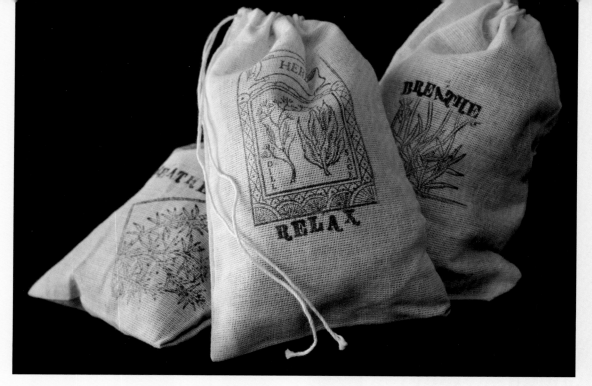

▪ Mint Sachets For the Car

Give yourself a mini spa moment during a crazy travel commute. Have stress-relieving squishy sachets filled with peppermint in your car. Someone cut you off in traffic? Stressed because you're late? Grab this sachet and squeeze it to release the fresh minty aroma. These make nice natural air fresheners to keep in the car.

Dried peppermint leaves
Muslin drawstring bags

What to do:

- ▪ Fill bags, draw the string and knot tightly to close.

FRAGRANT THERAPY

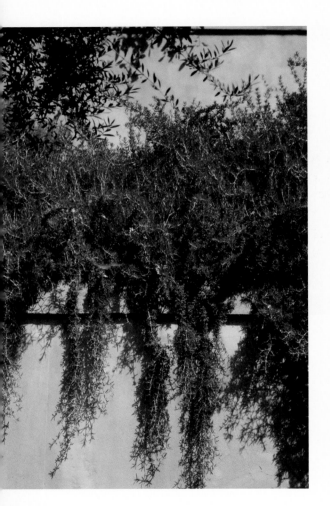

Aromatherapy is the use of fragrance for healing. The lure and power of fragrance is legendary, from the use of crushed fragrant plants in ancient history to the alternative therapies of the modern world. Scientists have recorded that there are several dozen emotional responses to flower scents. The power of fragrance can bring back pleasant memories as well as relax and uplift moods, all of which defines what "aromatherapy" really is. Heavily fragrant and oily plants have thick, volatile compounds that provide a protective layer around leaves. An English custom of covering garden walls with climbing rosemary for cooling has been supported by modern research. Rosemary has 74 times the cooling effect of fresh air due to its heavy fragrant nature.

Here are some ideas to capture the natural healing forces by blending herbs with other healing ingredients to target a specific need.

Lavender Healing Ointment

Excellent for soothing burned, chapped and scarred skin.

3 tablespoons grated beeswax
4 tablespoons sweet almond oil
3 teaspoons grated cocoa butter
10 drops Vitamin E oil
15 drops lavender essential oil

What to do:

- In a glass saucepan over low heat, slowly warm the beeswax, almond oil and cocoa butter until well combined. Remove from heat, allow to cool slightly.

- Add the Vitamin E and lavender oil. Mix well.

- Pour into jar and allow to cool down to a smooth balm texture. It will keep for 6 to 12 months.

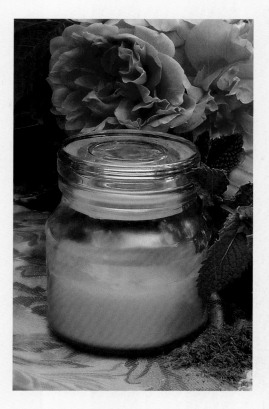

■ Cucumber Poultice

The common vegetable cucumber is a super skin healer. Combined with Aloe vera it becomes an amazing treatment. Use on sunburned and irritated skin to bring cooling relief.

1 fresh aloe vera leaf   **1 cucumber, organically grown**

What to do:

■ Peel skin off cucumber, split lengthwise and remove seeds. Crush or blend until it becomes become thick and pulpy.

■ Split the leaf of an Aloe vera and scrape the clear sap out with a spoon. Add the sap to the cucumber mush.

■ Apply to skin and allow to remain for up to 15 minutes. Rinse and pat dry. This be used repeatedly until burning and irritation subsides.

■ Ginger Tea Bath

Invigorating and healing in cold weather. Ginger stimulates and encourages skin to release toxins by promoting sweating. As the body recovers from sickness, this helpful bath will encourage the body to heal naturally.

¼ cup of fresh grated ginger   **2 cups water**
1 fresh lemon

What to do:

■ Bring water to a boil. Remove from heat and add grated ginger. Steep for 15 minutes.

■ Squeeze in the juice of one lemon. Mix well.

■ Pour the mix in a warm bath and soak for 10 to 15 minutes.

■ Double the recipe if you like to fill the tub to the rim.

Herbal Epsom Soak

Epsom salt has the ability to draw impurities out of the body. Use in the bathtub or as targeted soaks. Steep feet or other injured and inflamed areas such as elbows or wrist to relieve swelling.

1 cup Epsom salt
For a refreshing bath: **use 4 to 6 drops eucalyptus essential oil**
For a relaxing bath: **use 6 to 8 drops lavender essential oil**

What to do:
- In a small bowl, mix salt and essential oils together.

Thyme Astringent

Thyme has a natural antibacterial and cleansing property. When infused into liquid it becomes a usable form to wash skin. Use as a fragrant clean-up on hands, neck and face after a workout or busy day out in the garden pulling weeds.

½ cup distilled water   **½ cup vodka or witch hazel**
2 tablespoons fresh lemon thyme

What to do:
- Bring water to boil, remove from heat and cool slightly.
- Add lemon thyme and allow to steep in the water for about 15 minutes. The longer you allow the mix to sit, the stronger the infusion and fragrance.
- Filter out the remnants of thyme. Transfer to a clean, glass jar and add vodka or witch hazel. Keep refrigerated for a cool splash.

IN YOUR FACE

Nourish and clean for a fresh face experience. A facial forces you to slow down, because a facial stops you from multitasking. Add a sensual note to face time by giving a facial to a friend or loved one.

Exfoliate, mask, tone, moisturize. Make time for all the steps in one sitting to revitalize and give a healthy glow. The recipes and herbs below are for typical normal skin. Do this ultra-nourishing face treatment once a month.

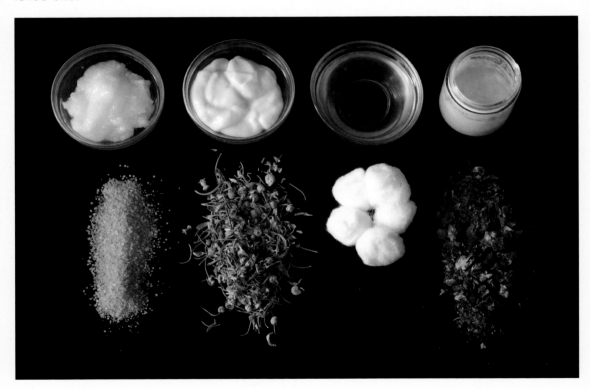

■ Step one: *Exfoliate*

This removes dead skin cells and toxins from the surface of the skin. Be very gentle and take it slow. Use calming circular motions, avoiding the eyes.

Sugar Coconut Scrub

1 cup sugar   ½ cup coconut oil

What to do:

- Mix well and use immediately.

■ Step two: *Mask*

Oatmeal and Herbs Mask

¼ cup whole oats   1 tablespoon dried rosemary leaves
¼ cup dried calendula petals   Plain yogurt or avocado
1 tablespoon dried Roman chamomile

What to do:

- Mix dry ingredients well and grind into a powder. This mix can be stored for later use as the herbal base to a fresh mask.

To use:

- Add 1 tablespoon of herb base to 1 tablespoon warmed plain yogurt or smashed avocado. Stir to mix well, adjust the amount of ingredients to achieve a nice spreadable consistency. Apply to face and relax for about 20 minutes. The mask will begin to tighten and dry as it draws out toxins.

■ Step three: *Tone*

Splash on this herbal toner to wash away traces of the exfoliated cleanser and tighten pores.

Chamomile Finishing Toner

2 cups distilled water
½ cup dried chamomile flowers

¼ cup organic apple cider vinegar
  or witch hazel extract (if the smell
  of vinegar is bothersome)

What to do:

- Warm the water (do not boil) and add the chamomile flowers. Remove from heat and allow to steep for 15 minutes.
- Add vinegar, mix well. Filter out the remnant herbs and discard.
- Store toner in a sterilized glass jar. The toner will store up to six months.

■ Step four: *Moisturize*

Finish the skin glow and seal in the moisture with this light, simple cream that won't clog pores.

Rosewater Cream

2 tablespoons sweet almond oil
3/4 tablespoon grated beeswax

1 tablespoon rosewater (purchased
  or homemade; recipe follows)

What to do:

- Combine beeswax and oil. Heat just until beeswax melts.
- Remove from heat and allow to cool.
- Stir in the rosewater and make sure ingredients are mixed well.
- Store in a glass bottle.

▪ Rosewater

You can purchase rosewater to use in spa treatments, but if you have access to fresh organic rose petals, it is easy to make small batches of your own. Use rose petals from organic roses that have just begun to open. The more fragrant the petals, the stronger the scent and properties of the rosewater. Pick them when they are at their prime and not over-aged.

½ to 1 cup fresh-picked, clean rose petals

2 cups distilled water

3 tablespoons vodka (used as a preservative)

What to do:

- Place clean rose petals in a sterilized glass jar. Add water and vodka to completely cover.

- Gently crush petals with a wooden spoon to help release the natural oils into the water mix. Cover and place in a warm area or sunny windowsill. Allow to sit for 2 weeks.

- Strain the used petals from the water and rebottle.

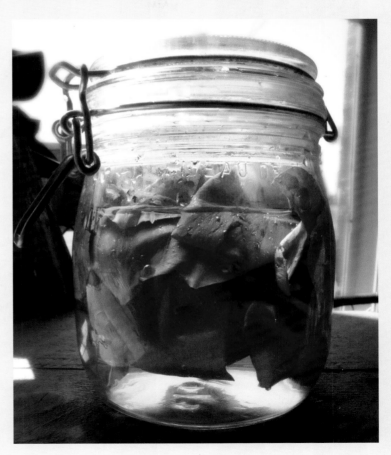

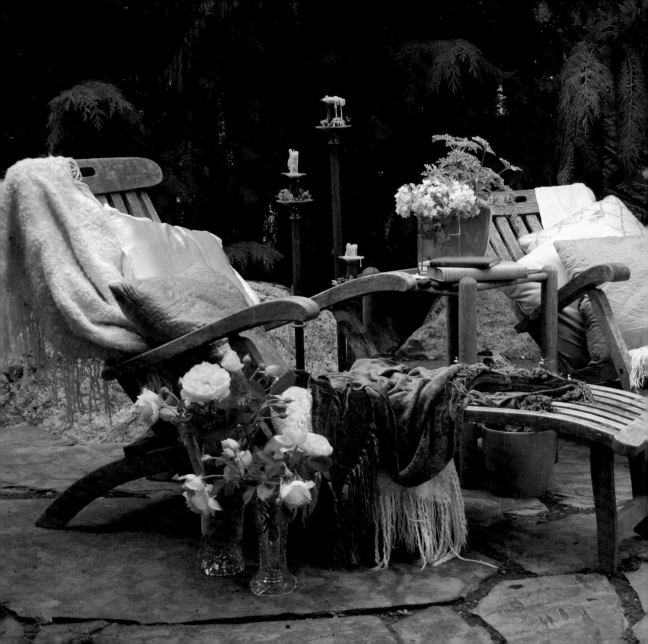

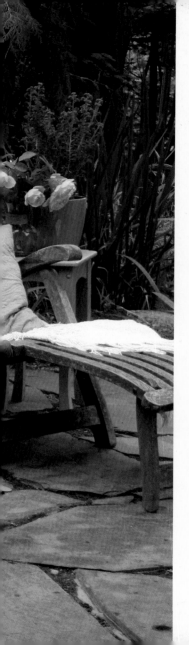

A MIDSUMMER'S EVE CELEBRATION

The summer solstice is the longest day of the year. Ancient celebrations paid homage to the light knowing from that point on, days would slowly become shorter. In the same time period Christianity celebrated a feast day for St. John the Baptist, which was the day after the summer solstice. Legend is woven with romantic and mystical tales of happenings on the longest day of the year. Whatever your mind conjures up over the stories, the enticement of the abundance of summer is reason enough to celebrate. You can walk through the garden and gather almost every herb at its peak, including the delicate blue borage flowers, lavender, mint, thyme, scented geranium leaves and calendula.

Immerse yourself in the lavishness of summer with the ultimate sensual summer spa. Make light, fragrant waters to mix with other ingredients like sea salt for scrubs or base oils for massage. Gather friends for a party! Offer herbal spritzers for drinking, hand and foot massage goodies that carry the freshness of a summer garden. Set a buffet table with spa treatments, a stack of hand and paper towels, give a quick how-to and ask guests to indulge.

▪ Floral Garden Water

A handful of fragrant, fresh rose
petals, plus additional handful
for later

2 tablespoons fresh lavender buds

A handful of fresh spearmint

2 cups pure filtered water

½ cup witch hazel or vodka
(optional as a preserver)

3 drop lavender essential oil,
if desired

3 drops rose essential oil, if desired

What to do:

- Bring water to boil in a glass pan,
  remove from heat.

- Add the lavender, spearmint and one
  handful of rose petals and allow to sit
  for 30 minutes. This will make a simple
  water infusion of the fragrant plants.

- Filter out the plants and add the
  second handful of fresh rose petals.

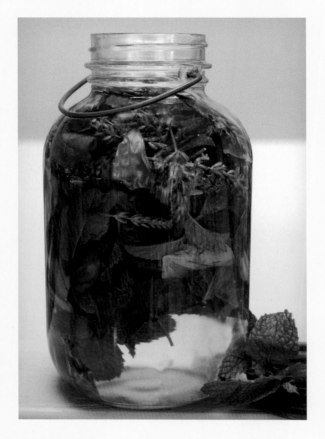

- Pour in the vodka or witch hazel (has a slight odor) and shake to mix well.

- Allow to sit in the sun for another 30 minutes. Strain off the plants through a coffee filter
  or cheesecloth.

- Add essential oil if desired and shake well. Pour into a glass bottle with a spray mister
  top. Shake well before each use.

◾ Floral Water Skin Brightener

½ cup floral water
¼ cup plain yogurt
1 tablespoon baking soda

What to do:

- ◾ Mix all ingredients until smooth. This should have a good creamy consistency, not watery or runny.
- ◾ Gently massage into damp skin in circular motions all over face and neck. Avoid tender eye areas. Rinse well.

Other Ways to Use Floral Waters

- ◾ Saturate a cotton ball and use as a face and neck wash.
- ◾ Mist hair and skin with scented water before going out for the evening.
- ◾ In a soaking tub, pour scented water and add a handful of fresh rose petals and lemon verbena leaves to float in the surface. If you are lucky to have an outdoor tub, this is the ultimate summer bath blend. All you need is candles and a warm, relaxing evening.
- ◾ Spray scented herbal waters onto linens to refresh them just before retiring for the night.
- ◾ Add 1 cup sweet almond oil to one cup floral water, shake well before use. After a shower or sauna treatment, coat skin from head to toe with this light fragrant mix.

Two refreshing summertime drinks to add to your party or spa time:

▪ Peach and Rosemary Spritzer

1 cup water

1 cup sugar

3 large peaches, peeled and sliced into small pieces

3 sprigs rosemary (use soft-stemmed pieces)

What to do:

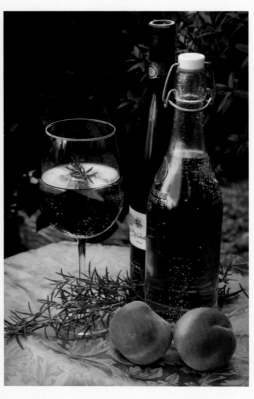

- Bring water to boil in a medium glass saucepan, add sugar and stir until dissolved, to create a sugar syrup.

- Stir in the peaches. Remove from heat and add rosemary. Cover and let cool completely.

- Remove rosemary sprigs and place syrup blend in a glass pitcher. Refrigerate at least 2 hours or overnight.

To serve:

- White wine spritzer: Pour ¼ cup of syrup into an 8-ounce glass; add ice cubes. Pour white wine until glass is about 3/4 full, top with club soda to add the "spritz." Garnish with a fresh peach slice and a sprig of fresh rosemary.

- Non-alcoholic spritzer: Pour ¼ cup of syrup in a glass, add ice cubes, and fill glass with club soda. Garnish with a fresh peach slice and a sprig of fresh rosemary.

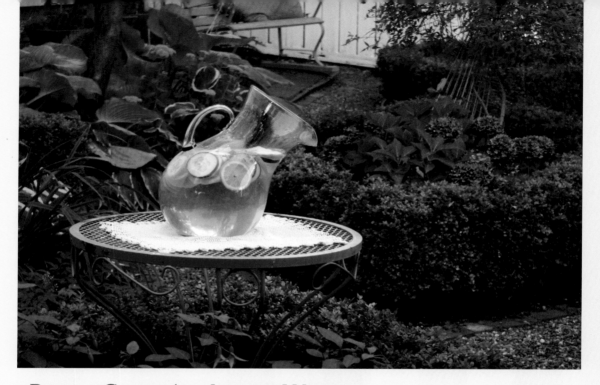

■ Borage Cucumber Lemon Water

A refreshing way to flavor drinking water.

1 organic cucumber,
  peeled and thinly sliced

2 lemons
Borage blossoms

What to do:

- Wash the outer skin of the lemons, slice and remove seeds.

- In a pitcher, fill about ¼ full of ice cubes. Add fresh water until almost full.

- Add cucumber, lemon, and float borage blossoms. Serve immediately.

▪ Dusty Rose Body Powder

2 to 3 fresh leaves of scented geranium
   (*Pelargonium* 'Attar of Roses' or *P.* 'Lady Plymouth')
¾ cup loosely packed fresh rose petals
½ cup cornstarch
½ cup white rice flour
10 drops rose geranium essential oil

What to do:

- Pat leaves and rose petals dry and allow to wilt overnight before adding to the powder mix.

- Mix together rice flour and cornstarch in a bowl.

- Place one geranium leaf in the bottom of a glass canning jar and just enough cornstarch/rice flour mix to cover the leaf. Add a layer of rose petals, top with cornstarch flour mix and alternate the layers until the jar is full. Cover and set aside for one week.

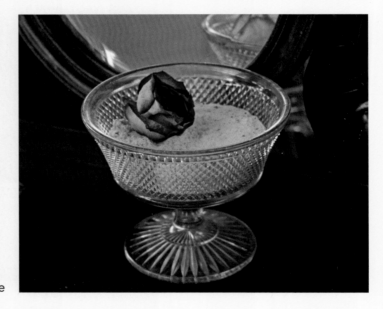

- Shake well. Sift out the rose petals and scented geranium leaves. Mix in rose geranium oil, stir well and place in a glass shaker jar.

WINTER SOLSTICE

The sun is lower in the sky and the darkness of evening sets in early. These are the days of winter. We wrap ourselves in warm blankets to shake off the cold. The garden reflects silhouettes of bare branches and the abundance of summer is hidden beneath the snow. In mid-December, the winter solstice marks when the day is the shortest and the sun begins its slow progress to give longer daylight. We become meditative, stay inside and feel like we want to hibernate. Relying on the herbs harvested and preserved from summer, skin treatments relieve dry skin. Bathing in herbs encourages positive meditation in this introspective time to spark a renewal as nature works her way to spring.

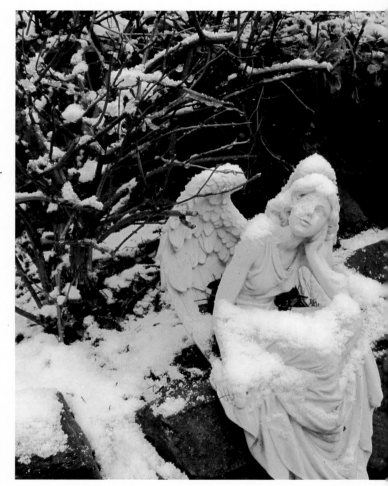

■ Calendula Salve

Healing and colorful, this salve is pure and simple to soothe hands, elbows, and rough patches of skin worn by the drying effects of indoor heat.

1 cup dried calendula petals
1 cup olive or avocado oil

1 tablespoon beeswax
1 Vitamin E capsule

What to do:

■ Pour the oil into a clean, sterilized glass jar. Add calendula petals to oil and snip floating petals to break up larger pieces.

■ Cover the jar and allow to sit for two weeks, shake occasionally.

■ *Optional:* You can speed up the process by warming the calendula petal/oil mix. Microwave for a minute or until the oil is warm (not burning hot). The heat will release the properties of the calendula into the oil. Allow to cool before use.

■ When the oil is ready, filter out the petals through a strainer or cheesecloth. Pierce the Vitamin E capsule and squeeze into the oil, mix well. Set aside.

■ Slowly melt beeswax in a glass saucepan over low heat, until fully liquefied. Remove from heat and slowly pour in the calendula oil, stirring until the mix is blended and just begins to harden.

■ Pour into small wide-mouthed tins or jars. Cover.

Salves, Balms and Solid Perfume: thick or thin?

Mixtures of oil with a wax can be made to different consistencies based on the ratio of oil to wax. If you are going to use the salve for hands, elbows, and as a lip balm, then more wax will be added. If it is used for massage or to be spread over a wider area, use more oil for a softer mix. If a blend is too solid after making a recipe, re-melt over low heat and add a small amount of oil. Add a few shavings of beeswax if it is too soft.

Simple Herb Soap

A 7-ounce bar of pure soap (glycerin, olive oil or other natural-based, non-fragrant soap)

1 tablespoon dried herb of choice

8 drops essential oil (the same as the chosen herb)

What to do:

- Finely grate the soap bar into small shavings with a cheese grater.

- Melt slowly over a double boiler on the stove until the soap becomes completely liquid (keep careful watch and never allow to boil or burn).

- Let cool slightly and stir in the remaining ingredients. Pour liquid mix into molds or roll into balls and allow to harden.

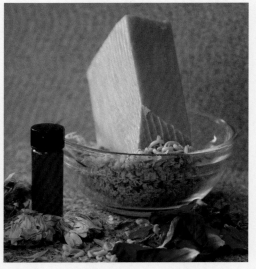

Soapy Herbs

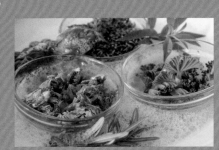

Choose the herbs for the qualities you want in a simple soap. All of these herbs blend well and add fragrance to the base soap.

Lavender: gentle and calming

Calendula: calming, adds a natural color

Rosemary: cleansing and antibacterial

Lemon verbena: healing and refreshing

Scented geranium: good for mature skin

Basil: rich clove-like aroma (Burgundy leaf basil varieties will infuse a dark red color)

▪ Winter Warming Steam

If you have a small bathroom, it makes an ideal space for this relaxing winter steam. Fill the air with the skin warming qualities of ginger, freshened with lemon.

1 teaspoon fresh grated ginger
1 fresh lemon

What to do:

▪ In a small bathroom, close the door. Roll up towels and cover the space between the floor and the door or any place the warmth might escape. This will help hold the aromatic steam in the room for a longer period of time. Fill the bathroom sink with very hot water. Float the ginger and sliced fresh lemon in the water and allow to permeate the room. Breathe deeply, sit and relax with a book or music to enjoy the benefits.

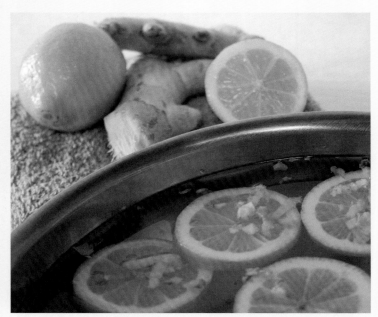

FURTHER
INFORMATION

■ ■ ■

GLOSSARY

RESOURCES

RECIPE LIST

INDEX

GLOSSARY of TERMS

Anti-inflammatory: reduces swelling and inflammation.

Anti-oxidant: inhibits the binding of oxygen. Prevents oxygen from damaging a living organism.

Astringent: will tighten and tingle skin. This creates a natural protection from outside elements.

Balm: oil infused with herbs, solidified with a natural wax and used as a lotion on skin.

Carrier: a term used to describe the base that herbs are infused into. It "carries" the herb to put it into a pourable, spreadable or other useable form. Water, alcohol, oil, vinegar are all types of carriers.

Carrier/Base oils: natural oils derived from plants, nuts or fruits. They typically have little or no smell. Commonly used in natural preparations to achieve a base or texture. The oils also contain their own natural healing properties. Use high quality, cold-pressed if available. Example: jojoba, safflower, sweet almond, avocado, wheat germ, vitamin E, apricot kernel, etc.

Decoction: an extraction method for tougher parts of herbs like bark, roots and seeds. To make: Place approximately 3 tablespoons of dried herb in a small saucepan. Cover herbs completely with 4 cups of cold water. Slowly heat the water until simmering, not a rolling boil. Simmer for 30 minutes. Allow to cool and strain out the herb, then bottle the liquid.

Emollient: an ingredient that maintains a smooth, soft, pliable appearance on skin.

Emulsifier: a natural ingredient that forces oil to disperse in water.

Exfoliant: an abrasive texture used to remove waste and dead cells from skin.

Humectant: a substance that prevents water loss on skin.

Infusion: a method of steeping herb leaves and flowers in water to extract the properties of the plant. Teas are typically made by infusion. To make: Heat 1 cup of water to a boil, remove from heat. In a glass mug or bowl, pour the boiling water over 1 to 2 teaspoons of herbs, cover and let stand for at least 15 minutes and as long as 30 minutes to release the properties of the herb into the water. Steep out and use fresh.

GLOSSARY of TERMS

pH: a measure from 1 to 14 of acidity and alkalinity. Seven (7) is neutral and a balance of both. Skin tends to be acidic at about 5.5 pH. The balance of oily or dry in skin care is based on what end of the pH scale it falls in. Soap tends to be alkaline (high pH) and that is why it dries out skin. Cleansers tend to have a higher pH to help break up oils and dirt. When a product says it restores pH, it helps bring the pH number down to skin's natural acidic level.

Poultice: a pulp made of herbs, fruit or vegetables that is typically applied directly to skin. To make: Chop or grind fresh herbs until they are sticky and oozing natural juice. For dry herbs, add fresh distilled water or the appropriate herb infusion or tincture to create the pulp.

Salve: a mix of oil and wax with herbs. Typically heavier in texture than a balm, salve is used for healing burns and skin irritations.

Steam distillation: a method of steaming plant material to release the essential oils.

Tincture: herbs in a liquid base ingredient, typically alcohol. Herbs infused in vodka or grain alcohol have a long shelf life. Dilute and use for a cleansing astringent and additions to floral waters. To make: Fill a clean, sterilized pint-size canning jar with fresh herbs. Pour vodka to the top of the jar. Cover and shake well. Allow to sit for up to 6 weeks. Shake jar occasionally. When liquid is heavily fragrant with the herb, strain out and store liquid in a tinted glass bottle.

Toner: prepared with ingredients that restore acidity to the skin after cleansing. They are made to tighten and close skin pores.

Wax: Natural waxes used to solidify preparations.

RESOURCES

Herbs, Oils and Supplies

Aura Cacia essential oils: 800-437-3301,
www.auracacia.com

Frontier Natural Products Co-op: 800-669-3275,
www.frontiercoop.com

Mountain Rose Herbs: 800-879-3337,
www.mountainroseherbs.com

Starwest Botanicals: 800-800-4372,
www.starwest-botanicals.com

The Essential Oil Company: 800-872-8772,
www.essentialoil.com

Packaging

SKS Bottle and Packaging: 519-880-6980,
www.sks-bottle.com

Sunburst Bottle: 877-925-4500,
www.sunburstbottle.com

Crochet Instruction and Information

www.craftyarncouncil.com

Plants and Seeds

Shop your local garden stores and farmers markets first!

Mountain Valley Growers: 559-338-2775,
www.mountainvalleygrowers.com

Nichols Garden Nursery: 800-422-3985,
www.nicholsgardennursery.com

Renee's Garden Seeds: 888-880-7228,
www.reneesgarden.com

Richter's Herbs: 905-640-6677,
www.richters.com

Territorial Seed Company: 800-626-0866,
www.territorialseed.com

Herb Publications

Herb Quarterly:
www.herbquarterly.com

Mother Earth News:
www.motherearthnews.com

Mother Earth Living:
www.motherearthliving.com

Herb Societies and Resources:

American Botanical Council:
www.herbalgram.org

Herb Research Foundation: www.herbs.org

Herb Society of America: www.herbsociety.org

International Herb Association: www.iherb.org

North Carolina State University:
www.ncherb.org

The Herb Growing and Marketing Network:
www. herbworld.com

RECIPES

Preserving
Herbal Ice Cubes

Get Steamy
Herb Steam Bundles
Lavender Heat Pillow
Mini Steam Sauna for the Face
Lemon Verbena Splash

The Ritual of Bathing
Basic Bath Brew
Inspiration Bath
Oatmeal Soak

Tea Time
Tub Tea
Fabric Tub Tea Bag sewing how-to
Lavender Green Tub Tea
Drinking Teas;
    Sweet, Minty and Soothing
    Tangy Touch of Citrus
    Floral Blend
    Earl Grey and Lavender
    Oolong and Lemon Balm
    Darjeeling and Rose Petals
    White Tea and Chamomile
Fresh Herbal Sun Tea
Loose Leaf Tea and Herbed Ice Tea

Down to Your Soles
Peppermint Foot Soak
Cooling Herbal Foot Powder
Sweet Feet Sugar Scrub

A Manly Herbal
Beard and Face Cleanser
Wisdom Toner and Aftershave
Witch Hazel Extract
Hand and Nail Butter

The Scrub Experience – Top to Bottom
Lavender Spa Salt Glow
Floral Sugar Scrub
Spa Cloth crochet how-to
Après-Scrub Skin Oil

Jet Lag
Sleep Pillows
On-the-Go Face Scrub
Chamomile Eye Soothers
Herbal Dry Shampoo

Mint to Be
Scalp Tingle Mint Shampoo
At-work Revivers
Minty Sachets for the Car

Fragrant Therapy
Lavender Healing Ointment
Cucumber Poultice
Ginger Tea Bath
Herbal Epsom Soak
Thyme Astringent

In Your Face
Exfoliate Face Scrub
Facial Mask
Chamomile Finishing Toner
Rosewater Cream
Rose Water

Midsummer's Eve Celebration
Midsummer's Eve Floral Garden Water
Floral Water Skin Brightener
Dusty Rose Body Powder
Peach and Rosemary Spritzer
Borage Cucumber Lemon Water

Winter Solstice
Calendula Salve
Simple Herb Soap
Winter Warming Steam

REFERENCES

A listing of sources used for reference in this writing, and some favorite books from my personal library that inspire me:

Aromatherapy, Daniele Ryman, Bantam Books, 1993.

Aromatherapy Massage, Clare Maxwell-Hudson, Dorling Kindersley Limited, 1994.

The Aromatherapy Trade Council: www.a-t-c.org.uk

The Art of Perfumery and the Methods of Obtaining the Odours of Plants, G.W. Septimus Piesse, Ph.D., F.C.S. London Longmans, Green and Co., Cornell University, 1879.

The Book of the Scented Garden, F.W Burbridge, John Lane, 1905.

Dictionary.com, Unabridged. Random House.

Duke University Library: www.library.duke.edu/rubenstein/scriptorium/eaa/ponds.html

"The Essence of Herbs," article by Harriet Flannery Phillips, *The Herb Companion,* January 1993.

Fragrance: the Story of Perfume from Cleopatra to Chanel, Edwin T. Morris, Charles Scribner's Sons, 1984.

Gardening with Herbs, Helen M. Fox, The Macmillan Company, 1933.

Henry IV, Part 1, William Shakespeare

The Herb Companion magazine: no longer being published, but my stack of back issues is a treasure.

"The Herbal Home Spa," article by Sue Goetz, *West Sound Home and Garden* magazine, November 2009.

Herbs to See, to Smell, to Taste, Susan Goetz, self-published, 1993.

In Love with Lavender, Susan Goetz, self-published, 2008.

A Modern Herbal, Mrs. M. Grieve F.R.H.S, Jonathan Cape Limited, revised edition 1973.

Saltworks: www.saltworks.us

Taking the Waters, Alev Lytle Croutier, Abbeville Press, 1992.

University of Maryland: http://umm.edu/health/medical-reference-guide/complementary-and-alternative-medicine-guide/herb/lemon-balm

U.S. National Library of Medicine: http://www.ncbi.nlm.nih.gov/pubmed/22612017, "The effects of lavender oil inhalation on emotional states, autonomic nervous system, and brain electrical activity."

Favorites from My Library

Crabtree & Evelyn Fragrant Herbal, Lesley Bremness, Bulfinch Press, 1998.

Dream Pillows and Love Potions, Jim Long, Long Creek Herbs, 1993.

Herbal Well Being, Joyce A. Wardwell, Colleen K Dodt, Greta Breedlove, Storey Publishing, 2002.

Herbs for Natural Beauty, Rosemary Gladstar, Storey Publishing, 1999.

Natural Beauty at Home, Janice Cox, Henry Holt and Company, Inc., 1995.

The Complete Book of Herbs, Lesley Bremness, Viking Penguin Inc., 1988.

The Herbal Body Book, Stephanie Tourles, Storey Publishing, 1994.

Clip Art

1,001 Floral Motifs and Ornamentals for Artists and Craftspeople, Dover Publications, Inc., 2013.

200 Illustrations from Gerard's Herbal, Dover Publications, Inc., 2005.

Plants and Flowers: 1,761 Illustrations for Artists and Designers, Dover Publications, Inc., 1992.

INDEX

ACKNOWLEDGMENTS

Thankful, appreciative, grateful: just a few of the many words that come to mind to express my debt of gratitude to those involved in this project. I start with those who encouraged the writing of the book. My circle of garden writer friends is many, but a special note of thanks goes to Marianne Binetti. It was years ago and another book, but you didn't stop encouraging me. Your sage advice and enthusiasm are never ending. Thank you to Debra Prinzing for reminding me that I still had an herb book that should be published, and literally taking me by the hand for an introduction to the family of St. Lynn's Press.

Thank you, Paul Kelly, for challenging me (in a good way). I have a multitude of words scribbled on notebook pages after our early phone conversations about this book. As I look back on those, I truly see your vison to bring out the good in your writers. You trusted me to run with it and then gave me over to your awesome team. Cathy Dees, my editor and also a patient and calming influence – you have been my cheerleader and word master with a consistent reminder with every edit to keep my voice and just write. You have a very special gift that keeps the writer's voice from getting lost in the process. Holly Rosborough, art director at St. Lynn's – from the moment I knew you would be working on my book I never worried. Your talent precedes you. Thank you for giving my words life on a page.

I consider it a joy and privilege to visit private gardens and I am grateful to all those who let me come in and take photos. I want to give special mention to Cher Maplestone and David Kenworthy, Mark and Cindy Harp, and Diane Names, who gave extra attention to their gardens and homes when they heard I was coming by. Beautiful gardens shown in this book also include Debra Prinzing's, Katie Padwick's, Bradley Huson's and those on open garden tours. Thank you to Jori Adkins for letting me pick herbs and photograph your lovely garden spaces that surround my studio.

Thank you to Pam Sturgill and her staff at American Design and also the studio space at Urban Garden Company for photo shooting opportunities.

A true gift of my business is to have awesome landscape design clients. Many patiently allowed me to be distracted away from their projects during a busy spring and summer season. To have a client say, "Get your book done and then do my landscape design," is a wonderful bonus.

I do have the best job and it is as much about the people I meet as their gardens I get to design.

Lastly, to my family, Dad and Joni, Mom and Joe and my daughters, Alyssa, Hayley and Courtney. Words are not enough, (cliché, I know) but your unending support renders me speechless. I count my blessings daily because I have the gift of all of you.

A SPECIAL NOTE OF PHOTO CREDIT

To Courtney Goetz:

I get to be your mom and brag about how talented you are, because that is what moms get to do. Now there are pieces of this book that show the world more of your talent. Thank you for all you did to bring the words in my head to photographs. You patiently let me fuss over whether a towel was folded correctly or an herb leaf was perky enough. Your artistic eye caught the details I couldn't see. I am grateful for the time you gave to this book and I share all of its visual beauty with you. ✒♥

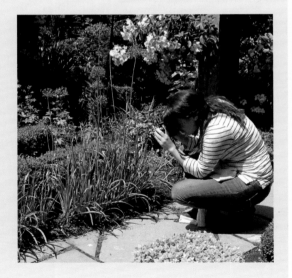

ABOUT THE AUTHOR

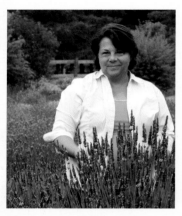

SUE GOETZ is a garden designer, writer and speaker. Through her garden design business, Creative Gardener, she works with clients to personalize garden spaces, from the seasonal tasks to the design of large projects. Her garden design work has earned many accolades: gold medals at the Northwest Flower & Garden Show, the Sunset Magazine Western Living award, the Fine Gardening Best Design award, and the AHS Environmental Award. Her home garden was featured in *Northwest Home and Garden* magazine, as well as *Country Gardens* magazine.

Writing and speaking are Sue's favorite ways to share her love of gardening. Her motto "...inspiring gardeners to create" defines all of her talks, with hands-on workshops, how-tos and ways to inspire creativity in and out of the garden. In 2012, she was named Educator of the Year by the Washington State Nursery and Landscape Association. Her work has appeared in numerous publications, including the *Tacoma News Tribune*, *Seattle Met*, *APLD Designer* magazine, *West Sound Home and Garden* and *Fine Gardening* magazine.

Sue is certified as a professional horticulturalist (CPH) with the WSNLA (Washington State Nursery and Landscape Association), and is a member of APLD (Association of Professional Landscape Designers), the Northwest Horticultural Society and The Garden Writers Association.

Sue lives and gardens in Washington State. She has three daughters who, no matter how far they roam, still call home for some of Mom's fragrant herbal concoctions.

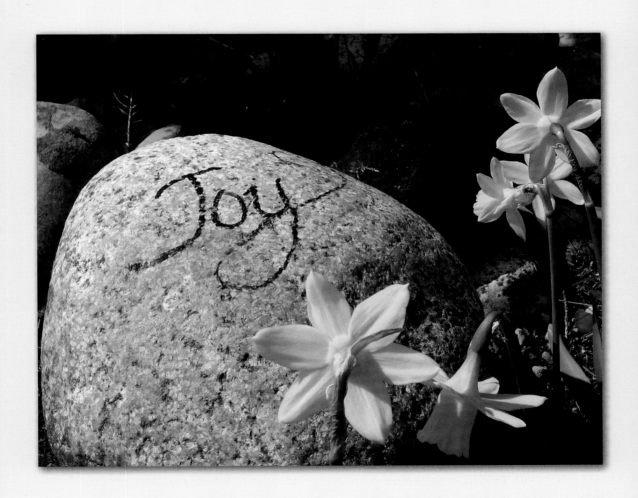

Other books from St. Lynn's Press

www.stlynnspress.com

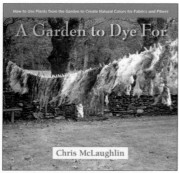

A Garden to Dye For
by Chris McLaughlin
160 pages, Hardback
ISBN: 978-0-9855622-8-1

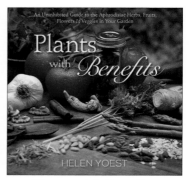

Plants with Benefits
by Helen Yoest
160 pages, Hardback
ISBN: 978-0-9892688-0-6

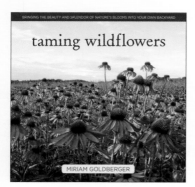

Taming Wildflowers
by Miriam Goldberger
208 pages, Hardback
ISBN: 978-0-9855622-6-7

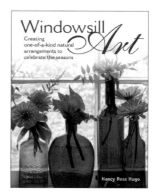

Windowsill Art
by Nancy Ross Hugo
192 pages, Paperback
ISBN: 978-0-9892688-5-1